T0140579

Cancer Drug Discovery and Development

Series Editor
Beverly A. Teicher

More information about this series at http://www.springer.com/series/7625

Amir R. Aref • David Barbie

Editors

Ex Vivo Engineering of the Tumor Microenvironment

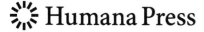 Humana Press

Editors
Amir R. Aref
Department of Medical Oncology
Dana-Farber Cancer Institute
Boston, MA, USA

David Barbie
Department of Medical Oncology
Dana-Farber Cancer Institute
Boston, MA, USA

ISSN 2196-9906   ISSN 2196-9914   (electronic)
Cancer Drug Discovery and Development
ISBN 978-3-319-83282-1   ISBN 978-3-319-45397-2   (eBook)
DOI 10.1007/978-3-319-45397-2

Printed on acid-free paper

This Humana Press imprint is published by Springer Nature
The registered company is Springer International Publishing AG
The registered company address is: Gewerbestrasse 11, 6330 Cham, Switzerland

To the memory of Morteza Salamat, my dear father in law, and Mrs. Sepideh Golzar, a wonderful friend who died of cancer during the preparation of this book in Iran.

Preface

While personalized or "precision" medicine is a major goal of cancer research, it has largely been relegated to the static measurement of genomic features, due to the inherent challenges of culturing tumors ex vivo. Recent major technological advances, however, have facilitated the ability to sustain the growth of primary tumor cells outside of the body, and to preserve and recapitulate features of the tumor microenvironment. Thus, it is now increasingly possible to expose patient-derived tumor samples to specific cancer therapies and measure responses to functional perturbations. In recognition of the growing potential of these technologies to advance the study of cancer biology and have a direct impact in the clinic, we felt it important to address the current state of patient-derived tumor models as they relate to the tumor microenvironment. We are thus pleased to provide *Ex Vivo Engineering of the Tumor Microenvironment* as a timely and comprehensive overview.

We want to sincerely thank all of the authors for their dedication and their outstanding contributions. We hope that you, as a reader, will enjoy this volume. A special thanks also goes to all of our dedicated colleagues at the Dana-Farber Cancer Institute who, with their tireless commitment toward cancer research, have become crucial factors in encouraging us to edit this book. We would also like to thank our families for their love and support. Finally, this work has ultimately been inspired by cancer patients themselves, especially those that have touched our own lives. We hope that by accelerating the development and application of these technologies, the day draws near that every individual that encounters this awful disease is cured.

Boston, MA, USA   Amir R. Aref, PhD
Fall 2016   David A. Barbie, MD

Contents

Introduction to Ex Vivo Cancer Models

Russell W. Jenkins

The field of cancer research has largely been guided by a reductionist focus on cancer cells and the genes within them—a focus that has produced an extraordinary body of knowledge. Looking forward in time, we believe that important new inroads will come from regarding tumors as complex tissues in which mutant cancer cells have conscripted and subverted normal cell types to serve as active collaborators in their neoplastic agenda. The interactions between the genetically altered malignant cells and these supporting coconspirators will prove critical to understanding cancer pathogenesis and to the development of novel, effective therapies.

—Hanahan and Weinberg, Cell 2000 [1]

1 Background: Opposing Views of the Cancer Universe

Cancer arises from acquired (and sometimes inherited) genetic changes in cells giving rise to a clonal population of neoplastic cells. However, continued growth of a tumor relies on recruitment and subversion of normal stromal elements [2]. In the cell autonomous view of cancer, a tumor is viewed primarily as a genetic disorder whereby a mutation (or series of mutations or other molecular changes) is sufficient to give rise to the malignant state. Thereafter, signaling transduction pathways become deranged, often in 'oncogene addicted' states that promote cell growth. In such states, transcriptional programs are co-opted to promote immortalization, resistance to cell senescence and apoptosis, escape of cell cycle checkpoints, promotion of growth of feeding blood vessels (angiogenesis), and ultimately adoption of an invasive and metastatic phenotype. This 'reductionist' view of cancer is in keeping with the original six hallmarks of cancer as detailed by Hanahan and Weinberg in 2000 [1]. This viewpoint is a useful construct and effectively

R.W. Jenkins (✉)
Department of Medical Oncology, Dana Farber Cancer Institute,
450 Brookline Avenue, Boston, MA 02215, USA
e-mail: rwjenkins@partners.org

© Springer International Publishing Switzerland 2017
A.R. Aref, D. Barbie (eds.), *Ex Vivo Engineering of the Tumor Microenvironment*,
Cancer Drug Discovery and Development, DOI 10.1007/978-3-319-45397-2_1

synthesizes decades of groundbreaking research to characterize the impact of oncogenic drivers and tumor suppressor genes in cancer cell biology.

The genomic era of medical oncology has arisen from the discovery that driver
mutations give rise to aberrant enzymes that promote cancer proliferation [1]. The
discovery of imatinib to target Bcr-Abl in chronic myeloid leukemia (CML) is often
cited as marking the beginning of the genomic era [3]. Over the last decade the
mutational landscape of multiple tumor types has been evaluated, and several cancers
are now sub-categorized based on the presence or absence of specific/targetable
driver mutations [4, 5]. Prior to the advent of the molecular era of cancer therapy,
these genetically aberrant cancer cells were targeted by cytotoxic chemotherapies—
the mainstay of cancer treatment—designed to derail the growth of these immortal
cells. While some cancers (e.g. lymphoma, testicular cancer, certain forms of leukemia) can be cured with chemotherapy, for most patients with advanced or metastatic
solid tumors (e.g. lung, breast, colon), the possibility of cure is unlikely and systemic treatment with chemotherapy is used to prolong life by months or years and/
or for palliative purposes (i.e. to reduce symptoms).

Following the discovery that various molecular abnormalities (i.e. mutations,
translocations, amplifications) defined specific cancers or cancer subsets, designer
drugs have been developed to target the abnormal proteins encoded by these mutant
genes. This notion of personalized medicine has offered great hope that curing cancer would be a matter of identifying the molecular abnormality driving a given cancer, and then designing a drug to inhibit this oncogenic protein. Small molecule
tyrosine kinase inhibitors (e.g. imatinib for Bcr-Abl) and monoclonal antibodies
(trastuzumab for Her2-amplified breast cancer) are capable of disrupting downstream signaling pathways in 'oncogene-addicted' cells, thereby restricting cell
growth and/or inducing cell death, and improving patient survival [3]. Advances in
molecular biology and genome sequencing technology have made next generation
sequencing of patient tumor samples readily available at most academic medical
centers. These technological advances along with the development of multi-
institutional collaborative efforts such as The Cancer Genome Atlas continue to
expand our knowledge of the diversity of molecular abnormalities in multiple cancers. This model has led to the identification of various driver mutations in several
cancers, including EGFR mutations [6] and anaplastic lymphoma kinase (ALK)
rearrangements [7] in non-small cell lung cancer, and BRAF mutations in melanoma
[8], which now have FDA-approved small molecule inhibitors as first line therapies.
Additional non-oncogene vulnerabilities [9] exist allowing targeting of specific cells
lineages rather than genetic alterations. Such therapies include anti-CD20 monoclonal antibodies (used in certain forms of lymphoma and leukemia) [10], as well as
Bruton's tyrosine kinase (BTK) inhibitors and PI3Kδ inhibitors, which have shown
dramatic efficacy in chronic lymphocytic leukemia (CLL) [11, 12].

Despite the promise of targeted therapies in certain molecular subsets of cancer,
clinical responses are often partial and/or short-lived [13]. While imatinib has
helped usher in the molecular era of cancer therapeutics, no targeted therapy has
been able to replicate the durable clinical responses seen in patients treated of
imatinib for chronic phase CML [3]. It is increasingly recognized that expanding

tumors become heterogeneous over time with various sub-clones emerging, especially under the selective pressure of targeted anti-cancer therapies [14–17]. Resistant clones can arise via multiple mechanisms, including mutations in the target enzyme, activation of bypass tracks, and gene amplification [18]. More recently, non-cell autonomous mechanisms involving dynamic interactions between cancer cells and non-neoplastic cells within the tumor microenvironment have been shown to foster the emergence of resistant cancer cells [19–22].

The *non-cell autonomous* (i.e. heterotypic) view of cancer incorporates other cell types into the cancer universe, and views cancer as a disease arising from complex network of biological interactions among and between multiple cell types. A cancer may arise from acquired somatic mutations, but these molecular alterations only serve to set the conditions for cancer development [22]. And while the cell autonomous effects of tumor mutations influence the phenotype of only the cells harboring those (epi)genetic changes, non-cell autonomous events are capable of influencing interaction between multiple cell types within the tumor microenvironment. During tumorigenesis there is a complex interplay between cancer cells and somatically non-mutated stromal elements, including immune cells, fibroblasts, and endothelial cells, and the sum of these interactions determines cancer growth and progression [2, 4]. These interactions involve intercellular communication via autocrine or paracrine signals, which can drive tumor growth [20, 21, 23] and resistance to anti-cancer therapies [22, 24], enhanced vascularization, matrix remodeling, and other pro-tumorigenic interactions within the tumor microenvironment. Many of these factors promote continued tumor growth, or resistance to therapy, through recruitment of stromal and immune cells that are co-opted and re-purposed to promote (rather than restrict) tumor growth [25, 26]. Incorporating the contribution of these non-cell autonomous effects into our view of cancer growth and response/resistance to therapy may provide a more accurate view of the natural dynamics of cancer growth in patients [4].

2 Preclinical Cancer Models: Of Mice and Men

Preclinical models are crucial for the study of cancer biology and for the rapid translation of key research findings into clinically useful therapies. Tools and techniques to model and study cancer have continued to evolve over the past decade. Current model systems include human-derived cancer cell lines and animal models of cancer. Cell culture using validated and standardized cancer cell lines has permitted remarkable advances in our understanding of cancer biology and was essential to usher in the molecular era of cancer investigation. Bolstered by animal, mostly murine, models of cancer and advances in our understanding of the cancer genome, there has been great hope that cancer could be cured simply by identifying the aberrant gene(s) and matching the right drug to the right patient.

Cancer cell lines grow easily in simple media, are relatively easy to propagate and genetically manipulate, grow readily on 2D culture surfaces, and can be used readily for drug screening, and can often grow in culture indefinitely [27]. Cancer cells grown in two-dimensional (2D) culture have been widely used by cancer biologists and pharmaceutical companies for routine drug screening and testing given their homogeneity and relative ease of culturing. The ability to interrogate multiple cell lines with dozens of drugs permits large-scale, high-throughput screening [28–32]. Large-scale characterization of dozens of cancer cell lines as part of a cancer cell line encyclopedia (CCLE) has been described as yet another system to model sensitivity of anti-cancer therapies using 2D culture of cancer cells [33]. Unfortunately, there are clear genetic, epigenetic, and transcriptional differences between cultured cells and native tumors in vivo [34], and the relevance of cancer cell lines as a model system to study complex cancer biology and for drug development has been called into question [27, 35].

Establishment of a permanent cancer cell line is not a trivial task, with reported success rates frequently less than 10%. Even when a cell line is successfully established investigation can be limited by the inherent absence of heterogeneity, inevitable genetic drift [27] leading to genetic and subsequently phenotypic instability [36–38]. Furthermore, in vitro growth of cancer cell lines on a plastic substratum has been shown to induce permanent changes in gene expression compared to growth as growth following implantation in immunocompromised mice [39]. Taken together, these issues raise fundamental questions about the ability of human cancer cell lines in 2D culture to accurately predict clinical efficacy of anti-cancer therapies.

Animal models of cancer have provided important insights into cancer biology that could not obtained from studying isolated cancer cell lines in vitro [40]. The overwhelming majority of animal studies use the laboratory mouse (*Mus musculus*) given the 99% overlap in genes, and genome that can readily be manipulated and engineered [41]. Mouse models of cancer include chemically induced carcinogenesis, xenografts, and genetically engineered models of cancer, all of which have proven powerful tools to evaluate complex tumor biology in a living organism [40, 42]. These mouse models have helped expand our understanding of cancer biology within a living organism, but suffer several shortcomings. Mouse models are expensive and labor intensive, and while they are able to recapitulate many features seen in human tumors, they are ill suited for large scale high-throughput screening of novel therapies.

Patient-derived xenografts (PDXs) represent a cancer model system whereby patient-derived explanted tumor tissue is implanted in an immunodeficient (e.g. athymic nude or NOD/SCID) mouse [43]. PDXs demonstrate improved genomic stability compared to human cancer cell lines [44], but suffer a high rate of failed implantation [45] and lack a functional immune system [46]. And despite the genomic (and stromal) stability that has been demonstrated for early passage PDXs (compared to in vitro growth) [39], concern remains regarding late genomic changes and alterations in the stromal environment (e.g. altered murine vs. human fibroblasts and endothelial cells) [47]. Ectopic and orthotopic engraftment methods for PDXs have been tested, with preference for orthotopic (same original anatomic site) to more closely mimic the native tumor microenvironment [41, 48, 49]. But perhaps most important is that conventional mouse models of cancer have failed to predict clinical efficacy of anti-cancer therapies in human clinical trials [30–32, 50, 51]. Such inconsistent results have led to the development of more sophisticated mouse models (e.g. GEMMs, PDXs) as well as interest in "co-clinical trials" for parallel evaluation of drug testing in humans and mice [41, 52].

Regardless of the model system used for pre-clinical drug development, testing and validation, we must face the fact that only a small percent of patients with advanced cancer have available targeted therapies currently [53]. The molecular era has brought us the promise of personalized medicine to match 'the right drug with the right patient' although 10 % or fewer of patients with cancer treated in the modern era will receive such 'targeted' treatments. And even for those patients treated with targeted therapies, the benefit is often short-lived or partial. The limitations of today's therapies highlight the need not only for better therapies, capable of providing long-term, durable disease control, but also for better preclinical cancer models that can provide a more clinically meaningful setting in which drug testing can occur. Durable disease control with targeted agents may be feasible with the drugs of tomorrow, but will require novel approaches to overcome the limitations of pre-clinical drug testing today.

3 Current and Future Approaches to Evaluate the Tumor Microenvironment

While the cell autonomous view of cancer has been essential to understand the contributions of individual oncogenic drivers and tumor suppressors, tumor heterogeneity, resistance programs, and tumor microevolution, it fails to address the complex interactions between these genetically abnormal cancer cells and the stromal components that we will hereafter to refer to as the *tumor microenvironment* (*TME*) [54]. Tumors are not simply collections of growing neoplastic cells, but rather are comprised of a complex microenvironment consisting of cancer cells as well as stromal and immune cells [55, 56]. The natural microenvironment in which tumors grow is a mixture of neoplastic cells along with supporting stromal elements, including immune cells, extracellular matrix (ECM), and blood and lymphatic vessels [57]. The interactions between multiple cell types, as well as interactions between cells and acellular elements of the TME is a complex and dynamic process [4, 58]. There is accumulating evidence that resistance to both targeted therapies and cytotoxic chemotherapies results from complex interactions with in the tumor microenvironment [59]. Roles for various stromal components in cancer progression (e.g. tumor-associated macrophages, cancer-associated fibroblasts, cancer-associated endothelial cells) have been described [4, 60, 61]. In recent years, the role of the immune system in both promoting and restricting tumor growth has become a topic of great interest [62, 63].

Oncology research is inherently translational given the goal of most (it not all) cancer research, whether directly or indirectly, is to identify effective therapies for patients suffering from cancer to improve quality of life (e.g. reduce symptoms), prolong life, or provide durable disease control or cure. The most widely used pre-clinical cancer model systems (as detailed above) are human cancer cell lines grown (in vitro) on artificial 2D surfaces and murine (in vivo) models. Due to the limited ability of 2D culture of cancer cells to recapitulate relevant features of the TME, this model system is less attractive, despite being a relatively easy and cost-effective way to screen novel compounds. Additionally, given the importance of immuno-therapy and immune checkpoint blockade as an emerging treatment modality to several cancer types, 2D growth of cancer cells is unable to address the involvement of the immune system in controlling tumor growth. Immunocompromised and immune-competent murine models exist, and can be employed to address the requirement for a functional immune system in the response to a given therapy. However, mouse models are time and labor-intensive, and quite costly and therefore often cost-prohibitive. Given the failure of most new drugs to provide substantial clinical benefit in phase III clinical testing, it has been suggested the failure of these investigational therapies may result (at least in part) from failure of preclinical mod-els to faithfully recapitulate human tumor biology [64], highlighting the need for new model systems.

Novel in vitro, ex vivo and in vivo cancer model systems have been developed recently with the goal of creating more relevant systems in which to study basic features of tumorigenesis, and to screen and test anti-cancer therapies [29]. Organoids [65], organotypic cultures [66, 67], circulating tumor cell-derived explants [68–71], and other ex vivo models using patient-derived tissue all have been suggested to serve as more clinically relevant model systems, to develop per-sonalized (tailored) treatment approaches [29, 72, 73].

Circulating tumor cells (CTCs) represent a very exciting modality to study the biology of cancer of dissemination and metastasis, but given their relative ease of collection from peripheral blood, there is great promise for functional evaluation of ex vivo drug response [69, 71, 74]. CTCs appear to grow better in suspension (as opposed to standard adherent culture), suggesting these cells exhibit biological fea-tures distinct from non-circulating cancer cells. Advances in microfluidic technol-ogy has offered another method for collection and study of CTCs, and there has been intense effort to scale up this technology for high-throughput analysis of drug libraries [74, 75]. However, while CTCs are clearly a very exciting source of patient-derived tissue, it can take months for the initial sample (often <100 cells) to be propagated in order to have sufficient cell numbers for such screening tests. Additionally, CTC cultures cannot currently address non-cell autonomous effects, given that only tumor cells are expanded and evaluated.

Conditional reprogramming (CR) technology, another method of propagating and manipulating patient-derived tumor samples ex vivo, involves growth of tumor samples in growth factor enriched media, an irradiated fibroblast feeder layer, and an inhibitor of Rho-associated protein kinase to induce an epigenetic state change [76, 77]. CR technology has been used to demonstrate the development of resis-tance to targeted therapies ex vivo using patient-derived samples, and also permitted identification of novel resistance mechanisms [78]. While this technology incorpo-rates patient-derived tissue into an engineered system to assess the long-term effects of drug exposure ex vivo, this system is still a 2D culture system that lacks an immune system. While likely an effective system for studying cell autonomous resistance to targeted agents, this system would require further adaptation to successfully model the native TME.

Organoids are human tissue surrogates derived from primary tissue (or stem cells) grown in vitro as a 3D multicellular clusters that are capable of self-organization and self-renewal [79]. They are generated by exposure of resected tumor tissue or biopsy samples to stem cell maintenance factors. To date, the greatest experience with cancer organoids has been limited to intestinally derived tumor types (e.g. colorectal cancer [80]), but more recently organoids have been generated from other cancer types, including prostate cancer [81] and pancreatic cancer [82]. Additionally, organoids are essentially pure epithelial cultures and lack a tumor stroma, vasculature, and immune cells, although involve interaction with a basement membrane (typically Matrigel®). Nevertheless, they provide a powerful tool to study early steps in carcinogenesis, interactions between normal epithelial cells and neoplastic cells, the role of cancer stem cells. Future studies will be needed to expand this technology to other cancer types and establish a broad collection of organoids for multiple cancer types that can be evaluated more extensively.

Organotypic cultures attempt to maintain the native stroma and tumor heterogeneity that is lacking in organoid culture systems, given both intra-patient tumor heterogeneity ("micro-diversity") and tumor-stromal interactions can influence cancer behavior and response to therapy [83, 84]. Such systems have included co-culture with multiple patient-derived cells lines, as well as culture of tumor slices using special culture plates and conditions [67] and heterogeneous tumor-derived spheroids (or "microspheroids") prepared by brief enzymatic and physical dissociation [73]. Multicellular tumor spheroids are aggregates of cancer cells that grow in 3D that more closely represent in vivo features of the tumor microenvironment [85]. Such systems that preserve the native TME can be used to profile ex vivo drug responses [72], and could be further adapted to study tumor-immune cells interactions in the TME [86].

Novel three-dimensional (3D) cancer model systems have been developed to provide a more realistic growth environment for cancer cells, often times with a model extracellular matrix [55]. Dynamic testing of drug sensitivity of cancer cells grown in 3D culture is emerging as an alternative to traditional 2D cell culture drug testing [87]. Drug sensitivity differs between cancer cell lines grown in 2D compared with cells or spheroids 3D continues to suggest that 3D culture systems may provide a more physiologically relevant system [88].

4 Opportunities and Future Directions

One of the greatest unmet needs in cancer biology is a model system to study interactions between tumor cells and the immune system [86], especially using primary human tumor samples. Decreased recognition by cytotoxic T lymphocytes, resistance to interferons, and impaired function of dendritic cells by tumor cells grown in 3D [89, 90] suggest that evaluation of interactions between cancer cells and the innate and adaptive immune systems in a 3D environment more closely represents the native environment in human tumors. This is a major limitation at present, but also represents an opportunity to engineer the next generation of ex vivo cancer model systems. The immune system has been shown to promote and restrict the growth of human cancers [91], but in recent years the activity of immune checkpoint inhibitory monoclonal antibodies targeting PD-1 and CTLA-4 has transformed the landscape of anti-cancer treatment options [63, 92]. Given the importance of the TME in influencing immune interactions, it is likely that the next generation of immune therapies will build on our understanding of immune stimulatory and inhibitory pathways to develop novel combination therapies to provide durable disease control to more and more patients [93]. In the meantime, existing ex vivo cancer models will continue to expand our knowledge of cancer biology with the hope of providing effective therapies to patients in need.

References

1. Hanahan D, Weinberg RA (2000) The hallmarks of cancer. Cell 100:57–70
2. Hanahan D, Coussens LM (2012) Accessories to the crime: functions of cells recruited to the tumor microenvironment. Cancer Cell 21:309–322
3. Druker BJ, Guilhot F, O'Brien SG, Gathmann I, Kantarjian H, Gattermann N et al (2006) Five-year follow-up of patients receiving imatinib for chronic myeloid leukemia. N Engl J Med 355:2408–2417
4. Hanahan D, Weinberg RA (2011) Hallmarks of cancer: the next generation. Cell 144:646–674
5. Lawrence MS, Stojanov P, Mermel CH, Robinson JT, Garraway LA, Golub TR et al (2014) Discovery and saturation analysis of cancer genes across 21 tumour types. Nature 505:495–501
6. Mok TS, Wu YL, Thongprasert S, Yang CH, Chu DT, Saijo N et al (2009) Gefitinib or carboplatin-paclitaxel in pulmonary adenocarcinoma. N Engl J Med 361:947–957
7. Kwak EL, Bang YJ, Camidge DR, Shaw AT, Solomon B, Maki RG et al (2010) Anaplastic lymphoma kinase inhibition in non-small-cell lung cancer. N Engl J Med 363:1693–1703
8. Flaherty KT, Puzanov I, Kim KB, Ribas A, McArthur GA, Sosman JA et al (2010) Inhibition of mutated, activated BRAF in metastatic melanoma. N Engl J Med 363:809–819
9. Luo J, Solimini NL, Elledge SJ (2009) Principles of cancer therapy: oncogene and non-oncogene addiction. Cell 136:823–837
10. Perez-Callejo D, Gonzalez-Rincon J, Sanchez A, Provencio M, Sanchez-Beato M (2015) Action and resistance of monoclonal CD20 antibodies therapy in B-cell Non-Hodgkin Lymphomas. Cancer Treat Rev 41:680–689
11. Cameron F, Sanford M (2014) Ibrutinib: first global approval. Drugs 74:263–271
12. Markham A (2014) Idelalisib: first global approval. Drugs 74:1701–1707
13. Holohan C, Van Schaeybroeck S, Longley DB, Johnston PG (2013) Cancer drug resistance: an evolving paradigm. Nat Rev Cancer 13:714–726
14. Marusyk A, Almendro V, Polyak K (2012) Intra-tumour heterogeneity: a looking glass for cancer? Nat Rev Cancer 12:323–334
15. Marusyk A, Polyak K (1805) Tumor heterogeneity: causes and consequences. Biochim Biophys Acta 2010:105–117

16. Michor F, Polyak K (2010) The origins and implications of intratumor heterogeneity. Cancer Prev Res (Phila) 3:1361–1364
17. Tabassum DP, Polyak K (2015) Tumorigenesis: it takes a village. Nat Rev Cancer 15:473–483
18. Wood KC (2015) Mapping the pathways of resistance to targeted therapies. Cancer Res 75:4247–4251
19. Marusyk A, Tabassum DP, Altrock PM, Almendro V, Michor F, Polyak K (2014) Non-cell-autonomous driving of tumour growth supports sub-clonal heterogeneity. Nature 514:54–58
20. Coppe JP, Patil CK, Rodier F, Sun Y, Munoz DP, Goldstein J et al (2008) Senescence-associated secretory phenotypes reveal cell-nonautonomous functions of oncogenic RAS and the p53 tumor suppressor. PLoS Biol 6:2853–2868
21. Kurtova AV, Xiao J, Mo Q, Pazhanisamy S, Krasnow R, Lerner SP et al (2015) Blocking PGE2-induced tumour repopulation abrogates bladder cancer chemoresistance. Nature 517:209–213
22. Tissot T, Ujvari B, Solary E, Lassus P, Roche B, Thomas F (1865) Do cell-autonomous and non-cell-autonomous effects drive the structure of tumor ecosystems? Biochim Biophys Acta 2016:147–154
23. Jouanneau J, Moens G, Bourgeois Y, Poupon MF, Thiery JP (1994) A minority of carcinoma cells producing acidic fibroblast growth factor induces a community effect for tumor progression. Proc Natl Acad Sci U S A 91:286–290
24. Obenauf AC, Zou Y, Ji AL, Vanharanta S, Shu W, Shi H et al (2015) Therapy-induced tumour secretomes promote resistance and tumour progression. Nature 520:368–372
25. de Visser KE, Eichten A, Coussens LM (2006) Paradoxical roles of the immune system during cancer development. Nat Rev Cancer 6:24–37
26. Mueller MM, Fusenig NE (2004) Friends or foes—bipolar effects of the tumour stroma in cancer. Nat Rev Cancer 4:839–849
27. Masters JR (2000) Human cancer cell lines: fact and fantasy. Nat Rev Mol Cell Biol 1:233–236
28. Friedman AA, Amzallag A, Pruteanu-Malinici I, Baniya S, Cooper ZA, Piris A et al (2015) Landscape of targeted anti-cancer drug synergies in melanoma identifies a novel BRAF-VEGFR/PDGFR combination treatment. PLoS One 10, e0140310
29. Friedman AA, Letai A, Fisher DE, Flaherty KT (2015) Precision medicine for cancer with next-generation functional diagnostics. Nat Rev Cancer 15:747–756
30. Johnson JI, Decker S, Zaharevitz D, Rubinstein LV, Venditti JM, Schepartz S et al (2001) Relationships between drug activity in NCI preclinical in vitro and in vivo models and early clinical trials. Br J Cancer 84:1424–1431
31. Takimoto CH (2001) Why drugs fail: of mice and men revisited. Clin Cancer Res 7:229–230
32. Talmadge JE, Singh RK, Fidler IJ, Raz A (2007) Murine models to evaluate novel and conventional therapeutic strategies for cancer. Am J Pathol 170:793–804
33. Barretina J, Caponigro G, Stransky N, Venkatesan K, Margolin AA, Kim S et al (2012) The cancer cell line encyclopedia enables predictive modelling of anticancer drug sensitivity. Nature 483:603–607
34. van Staveren WC, Solis DY, Hebrant A, Detours V, Dumont JE, Maenhaut C (1795) Human cancer cell lines: experimental models for cancer cells in situ? for cancer stem cells? Biochim Biophys Acta 2009:92–103
35. Lacroix M, Leclercq G (2004) Relevance of breast cancer cell lines as models for breast tumours: an update. Breast Cancer Res Treat 83:249–289
36. Engelholm SA, Vindelov LL, Spang-Thomsen M, Brunner N, Tommerup N, Nielsen MH et al (1985) Genetic instability of cell lines derived from a single human small cell carcinoma of the lung. Eur J Cancer Clin Oncol 21:815–824
37. Hausser HJ, Brenner RE (2005) Phenotypic instability of Saos-2 cells in long-term culture. Biochem Biophys Res Commun 333:216–222
38. Nielsen KV, Madsen MW, Briand P (1994) In vitro karyotype evolution and cytogenetic instability in the non-tumorigenic human breast epithelial cell line HMT-3522. Cancer Genet Cytogenet 78:189–199

39. Daniel VC, Marchionni L, Hierman JS, Rhodes JT, Devereux WL, Rudin CM et al (2009) A primary xenograft model of small-cell lung cancer reveals irreversible changes in gene expression imposed by culture in vitro. Cancer Res 69:3364–3373

40. Frese KK, Tuveson DA (2007) Maximizing mouse cancer models. Nat Rev Cancer 7:645–658

41. Herter-Sprie GS, Kung AL, Wong KK (2013) New cast for a new era: preclinical cancer drug development revisited. J Clin Invest 123:3639–3645

42. Cheon DJ, Orsulic S (2011) Mouse models of cancer. Annu Rev Pathol 6:95–119

43. Jin K, Teng L, Shen Y, He K, Xu Z, Li G (2010) Patient-derived human tumour tissue xenografts in immunodeficient mice: a systematic review. Clin Transl Oncol 12:473–480

44. Monsma DJ, Monks NR, Cherba DM, Dylewski D, Eugster E, Jahn H et al (2012) Genomic characterization of explant tumorgraft models derived from fresh patient tumor tissue. J Transl Med 10:125

45. Garber K (2009) From human to mouse and back: 'tumorgraft' models surge in popularity. J Natl Cancer Inst 101:6–8

46. Cutz JC, Guan J, Bayani J, Yoshimoto M, Xue H, Sutcliffe M et al (2006) Establishment in severe combined immunodeficiency mice of subrenal capsule xenografts and transplantable tumor lines from a variety of primary human lung cancers: potential models for studying tumor progression-related changes. Clin Cancer Res 12:4043–4054

47. Tentler JJ, Tan AC, Weekes CD, Jimeno A, Leong S, Pitts TM et al (2012) Patient-derived tumour xenografts as models for oncology drug development. Nat Rev Clin Oncol 9:338–350

48. Suetsugu A, Katz M, Fleming J, Truty M, Thomas R, Saji S et al (2012) Imageable fluorescent metastasis resulting in transgenic GFP mice orthotopically implanted with human-patient primary pancreatic cancer specimens. Anticancer Res 32:1175–1180

49. Waters DJ, Janovitz EB, Chan TC (1995) Spontaneous metastasis of PC-3 cells in athymic mice after implantation in orthotopic or ectopic microenvironments. Prostate 26:227–234

50. Day CP, Carter J, Bonomi C, Hollingshead M, Merlino G (2012) Preclinical therapeutic response of residual metastatic disease is distinct from its primary tumor of origin. Int J Cancer 130:190–199

51. Voskoglou-Nomikos T, Pater JL, Seymour L (2003) Clinical predictive value of the in vitro cell line, human xenograft, and mouse allograft preclinical cancer models. Clin Cancer Res 9:4227–4239

52. Chen Z, Cheng K, Walton Z, Wang Y, Ebi H, Shimamura T et al (2012) A murine lung cancer co-clinical trial identifies genetic modifiers of therapeutic response. Nature 483:613–617

53. Dienstmann R, Jang IS, Bot B, Friend S, Guinney J (2015) Database of genomic biomarkers for cancer drugs and clinical targetability in solid tumors. Cancer Discov 5:118–123

54. Whiteside TL (2008) The tumor microenvironment and its role in promoting tumor growth. Oncogene 27:5904–5912

55. Baker BM, Chen CS (2012) Deconstructing the third dimension: how 3D culture microenvironments alter cellular cues. J Cell Sci 125:3015–3024

56. Villanueva J, Herlyn M (2008) Melanoma and the tumor microenvironment. Curr Oncol Rep 10:439–446

57. Bissell MJ, Radisky D (2001) Putting tumours in context. Nat Rev Cancer 1:46–54

58. Tlsty TD, Coussens LM (2006) Tumor stroma and regulation of cancer development. Annu Rev Pathol 1:119–150

59. Chen F, Zhuang X, Lin L, Yu P, Wang Y, Shi Y et al (2015) New horizons in tumor microenvironment biology: challenges and opportunities. BMC Med 13:45

60. Mantovani A, Allavena P, Sica A, Balkwill F (2008) Cancer-related inflammation. Nature 454:436–444

61. Colotta F, Allavena P, Sica A, Garlanda C, Mantovani A (2009) Cancer-related inflammation, the seventh hallmark of cancer: links to genetic instability. Carcinogenesis 30:1073–1081

62. Fridman WH, Pages F, Sautes-Fridman C, Galon J (2012) The immune contexture in human tumours: impact on clinical outcome. Nat Rev Cancer 12:298–306

63. Pardoll DM (2012) The blockade of immune checkpoints in cancer immunotherapy. Nat Rev Cancer 12:252–264

64. Kamb A (2005) What's wrong with our cancer models? Nat Rev Drug Discov 4:161–165
65. Sachs N, Clevers H (2014) Organoid cultures for the analysis of cancer phenotypes. Curr Opin Genet Dev 24:68–73
66. Kenny HA, Lal-Nag M, White EA, Shen M, Chiang CY, Mitra AK et al (2015) Quantitative high throughput screening using a primary human three-dimensional organotypic culture predicts in vivo efficacy. Nat Commun 6:6220
67. Vaira V, Fedele G, Pyne S, Fasoli E, Zadra G, Bailey D et al (2010) Preclinical model of organotypic culture for pharmacodynamic profiling of human tumors. Proc Natl Acad Sci U S A 107:8352–8356
68. Baccelli I, Schneeweiss A, Riethdorf S, Stenzinger A, Schillert A, Vogel V et al (2013) Identification of a population of blood circulating tumor cells from breast cancer patients that initiates metastasis in a xenograft assay. Nat Biotechnol 31:539–544
69. Hodgkinson CL, Morrow CJ, Li Y, Metcalf RL, Rothwell DG, Trapani F et al (2014) Tumorigenicity and genetic profiling of circulating tumor cells in small-cell lung cancer. Nat Med 20:897–903
70. Yu J, Zhou X, Chang M, Nakaya M, Chang JH, Xiao Y et al (2015) Regulation of T-cell activation and migration by the kinase TBK1 during neuroinflammation. Nat Commun 6:6074
71. Zhang L, Ridgway LD, Wetzel MD, Ngo J, Yin W, Kumar D et al (2013) The identification and characterization of breast cancer CTCs competent for brain metastasis. Sci Transl Med 5:180ra48
72. Majumder B, Baraneedharan U, Thiyagarajan S, Radhakrishnan P, Narasimhan H, Dhandapani M et al (2015) Predicting clinical response to anticancer drugs using an ex vivo platform that captures tumour heterogeneity. Nat Commun 6:6169
73. Nagourney RA, Blitzer JB, Shuman RL, Asciuto TJ, Deo EA, Paulsen M et al (2012) Functional profiling to select chemotherapy in untreated, advanced or metastatic non-small cell lung cancer. Anticancer Res 32:4453–4460
74. Yu M, Bardia A, Aceto N, Bersani F, Madden MW, Donaldson MC et al (2014) Cancer therapy. Ex vivo culture of circulating breast tumor cells for individualized testing of drug susceptibility. Science 345:216–220
75. Brouzes E, Medkova M, Savenelli N, Marran D, Twardowski M, Hutchison JB et al (2009) Droplet microfluidic technology for single-cell high-throughput screening. Proc Natl Acad Sci U S A 106:14195–14200
76. Liu X, Ory V, Chapman S, Yuan H, Albanese C, Kallakury B et al (2012) ROCK inhibitor and feeder cells induce the conditional reprogramming of epithelial cells. Am J Pathol 180:599–607
77. Suprynowicz FA, Upadhyay G, Krawczyk E, Kramer SC, Hebert JD, Liu X et al (2012) Conditionally reprogrammed cells represent a stem-like state of adult epithelial cells. Proc Natl Acad Sci U S A 109:20035–20040
78. Crystal AS, Shaw AT, Sequist LV, Friboulet L, Niederst MJ, Lockerman EL et al (2014) Patient-derived models of acquired resistance can identify effective drug combinations for cancer. Science 346:1480–1486
79. Fatehullah A, Tan SH, Barker N (2016) Organoids as an in vitro model of human development and disease. Nat Cell Biol 18:246–254
80. Sato T, Stange DE, Ferrante M, Vries RG, Van Es JH, Van den Brink S et al (2011) Long-term expansion of epithelial organoids from human colon, adenoma, adenocarcinoma, and Barrett's epithelium. Gastroenterology 141:1762–1772
81. Gao D, Vela I, Sboner A, Iaquinta PJ, Karthaus WR, Gopalan A et al (2014) Organoid cultures derived from patients with advanced prostate cancer. Cell 159:176–187
82. Boj SF, Hwang CI, Baker LA, Chio II, Engle DD, Corbo V et al (2015) Organoid models of human and mouse ductal pancreatic cancer. Cell 160:324–338
83. Mengelbier LH, Karlsson J, Lindgren D, Valind A, Lilljebjorn H, Jansson C et al (2015) Intratumoral genome diversity parallels progression and predicts outcome in pediatric cancer. Nat Commun 6:6125
84. Junttila MR, de Sauvage FJ (2013) Influence of tumour micro-environment heterogeneity on therapeutic response. Nature 501:346–354

85. Sutherland RM (1988) Cell and environment interactions in tumor microregions: the multicell spheroid model. Science 240:177–184
86. Hirt C, Papadimitropoulos A, Mele V, Muraro MG, Mengus C, Iezzi G et al (2014) "In vitro" 3D models of tumor-immune system interaction. Adv Drug Deliv Rev 79–80:145–154
87. Ferrarini M, Steimberg N, Ponzoni M, Belloni D, Berenzi A, Girlanda S et al (2013) Ex-vivo dynamic 3-D culture of human tissues in the RCCS bioreactor allows the study of Multiple Myeloma biology and response to therapy. PLoS One 8, e71613
88. Ekert JE, Johnson K, Strake B, Pardinas J, Jarantow S, Perkinson R et al (2014) Three-dimensional lung tumor microenvironment modulates therapeutic compound responsiveness in vitro—implication for drug development. PLoS One 9, e92248
89. Feder-Mengus C, Ghosh S, Reschner A, Martin I, Spagnoli GC (2008) New dimensions in tumor immunology: what does 3D culture reveal? Trends Mol Med 14:333–340
90. Feder-Mengus C, Ghosh S, Weber WP, Wyler S, Zajac P, Terracciano L et al (2007) Multiple mechanisms underlie defective recognition of melanoma cells cultured in three-dimensional architectures by antigen-specific cytotoxic T lymphocytes. Br J Cancer 96:1072–1082
91. Palucka AK, Coussens LM (2016) The basis of oncoimmunology. Cell 164:1233–1247
92. Sharma P, Allison JP (2015) The future of immune checkpoint therapy. Science 348:56–61
93. Smyth MJ, Ngiow SF, Ribas A, Teng MW (2016) Combination cancer immunotherapies tailored to the tumour microenvironment. Nat Rev Clin Oncol 13:143–158

Patient-Derived Xenografts in Oncology

Dennis O. Adeegbe and Yan Liu

1 Introduction

Cancer is among the leading causes of death worldwide. In 2012, approximately 14 million new cases and about eight million cancer-related deaths were reported. In the United States, it is estimated that approximately 1,685,210 new cases of cancer will be diagnosed and 595,690 people will die from the disease (www.cancer.gov). Scientists for many years have been investigating cancer biology in an attempt to understand its development, mechanisms of progression and identify therapeutic agents to treat malignancies arising from various tissues. Animal models have long been used to investigate cancer biology providing an avenue to explore therapeutic efficacy of anti-cancer drugs and/or contribution of the immune system to tumor immunity. There are many models, ranging from in vitro culture systems utilizing human cell lines, to genetically engineered mouse models harboring specific genetic alterations, to mouse allograft models, to patient-derived xenograft (PDX) models. These existing investigational platforms vary in terms of their potential to recapitulate cancer biology as seen in patients [1, 2].

1.1 Generation of PDX Models (PDX Defined)

Patient-derived xenografts as the name suggests (PDX) encompasses the process of developing and maintaining (tumor) tissue obtained from a cancer patient an which is introduced into a secondary recipient host such as immunodeficient mice or rats typically by direct implantation of the human tumor cells. The source of tumor cells could

D.O. Adeegbe (✉) • Y. Liu
Medical Oncology, Dana Farber Cancer Institute,
450 Brookline Avenue, Boston, MA 02130, USA
e-mail: dennis_adeegbe@dfci.harvard.edu; yan_liu@dfci.harvard.edu

© Springer International Publishing Switzerland 2017

A.R. Aref, D. Barbie (eds.), *Ex Vivo Engineering of the Tumor Microenvironment*,
Cancer Drug Discovery and Development, DOI 10.1007/978-3-319-45397-2_2

be cell lines derived from human tumors after repeated cultures in vitro, fresh human tumor tissue obtained during re-sectioning surgery or biopsy either from primary site or metastatic lesions, tumor cells collected from malignant ascites or from blood, or tumor cell suspension after disaggregating the whole tumor. In the case of whole intact tumor tissue, this is often cut into small pieces of about 3–8 mm^3 prior to implantation. Upon engraftment of tumors in the first cohort (often termed F_0) of recipient mice, the growing tumors are removed and serially grafted onto another cohort over several passages (from $F_1 \cdots$ to F_n). Use of patient undissociated tumor specimen is considered to be superior in terms of overall tumor engraftment rate or "tumor take," an observation that could be attributed to the preservation of the tumor architecture and clonal population within the tumor [3]. Engraftment rates vary considerably between different models and different cancer types ranging from 25 to 100% [3]. Section 1.1.1 provides a general step-wise protocol for developing a standard PDX in immunodeficient NSG mice using fresh human cancer specimen and Fig. 1 provides a simplistic pictorial explanation of the basic process involved in establishing a PDX model.

Recipient mice commonly used in PDX models are the athymic nude which lack T cells but still have quantifiable adaptive immune system. More stringent than nude mice are the SCID and RAG2 knock out (KO) mice which are generally devoid of lymphocytes that make up the bulk of the adaptive immune system. With the

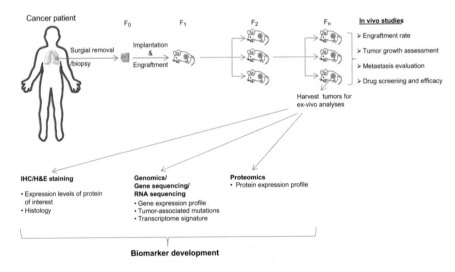

Fig. 1 Patient-derived xenograft establishment, propagation, and utility. Tumor specimen obtained from consented cancer patient undergoing surgery or biopsy is implanted unfragmented or dissociated into cell suspension and subsequently implanted either heterotopically or orthotopically into immunodeficient mice. Upon engraftment, tumor is excised surgically from the first cohort of recipient mice (F_1) and serially propagated over a number of passages in vivo ($F_2 \ldots Fn$). Tumor growth properties including engraftment rate and metastasis are evaluated often as part of drug screening and efficacy evaluation studies. Well established tumor grafts can be harvested for ex-vivo studies including immunohistochemistry, H&E staining, genomic studies, DNA and RNA sequencing, and proteomics

demonstrated contribution of NK cells to tumor immunity [4], other models lacking these cells such as the NOD.SCID and NOD.SCID IL-2Rγ KO mice have provided in vivo models considered to be most immunodeficient so far [5–7]. These mice are increasingly being used in both academic and industry-based drug research settings to conduct drug evaluation studies against cancer cells in PDX models. The benefits of these super immunodeficient mice is that they allow for greater tumor engraft-ment rates ranging from 90 to 100% and are particularly useful for tumors that are difficult to engraft and tumor-associated leukocyte subsets such as effector memory cells can persist in these hosts for up to 9 weeks after tumor implantation thereby allowing for studying tumor-immune cell cross talks [8].

How PDX implantation is performed differs from cancer types and/or sub-types. Specifically, site of implantation varies and can be heterotopic or orthotopic. Orthotopic simply means implantation at the tissue corresponding to that from which the tumor developed in a patient thereby allowing for studying the behavior of the tumor in its "natural" environment. Heterotopic on the other hand, is any site other than the ortho-topic location such as sub-cutaneous (s.c.) or under the renal capsule (sub-renal). The sub-renal implantation method is generally considered better than s.c. transplant model which is typically performed on the dorsal side of the mouse for a number of reasons: (a) engraftment rate is better and tumor architecture is better preserved, (b) most tumor-associated stroma is present at least initially, and most importantly, (c) the tumor genotype and phenotype is closer to the original tumor than tumor of s.c. PDX tumor. The choice of implantation site differs based on cancer types and/or sub-types and var-ies by investigator. Thus, the tissue of interest could be implanted either sub-cutane-ously, sub-renally, or orthotopically. While the former is easier to perform from a technical standpoint, the growth behavior of the implanted tumor may mirror that seen in the patient less well than the orthotopic approach. This would especially be critical for cancer types which derive additional support from the native surrounding tissue.

The number of passages that implanted tumors undergo is also critical to the architecture and overall biology of the cancer cells. It is generally recommended not exceed 5–6 passages as changes in gene expression pattern, gene copy numbers, and chromosomal stability may be altered considerably enough to change the morphol-ogy and genetic landscape of the grafts making these parameters divergent from the parental tumor [9–15]. As demonstrated in a number of reports, at low passages, gene expression profiles, histology, and chromosomal stability do not change con-siderably between the tumor graft and the parent tumor [16–19]. However, the pos-sibility exists that divergent changes may occur with increasing passages and this may be dependent on cancer type/sub-type and genotype. For instance, unlike colorectal PDX tumors with wild type p53 gene, those harboring mutant p53 gene underwent considerable chromosomal changes after several passages [17]. In con-trast, genomic alterations were infrequent in a breast cancer PDX model upon pas-sages spanning 2 ½ years [19]. While pancreatic PDX models passaged for up to 39 times revealed only modest genetic alterations [20]. In general, early passage tumors are used for drug treatment studies and there is no cut-off point per say as to which passage is most ideal. For the most part, the general consensus is that the less divergent the PDX tumor is in terms of histology and genetic landscape, the better for ascertaining its clinical relevance.

There are a number of other manipulations that can be performed to the input specimen prior to implantation depending on the aim of the study and endpoints. For example, small tumor pieces or single-cell suspensions can be mixed or coated with matrigel before performing the tissue graft. Other variations of standard PDX include mixing the tumor preparation with cells such as human fibroblasts, mesenchymal stem cells, etc. in an attempt to provide accompanying stromal components of human origin. Regardless of the PDX variation employed, the factors discussed above coupled with tumor type and precision of implantation are considerations that could impact the success of a PDX system and the overall behavior of engrafted tumor.

1.1.1 Materials

- Freshly excised tumor specimens, removed from a patient and stored in RPMI1640/1 % penicillin-streptomycin (Invitrogen 11875-093/15070-063) in a 50-ml conical tube at 4 °C for less than 24 h
- Optional; matrigel basement membrane matrix (BD Biosciences, 356237)
- NSG female mice at 4–6 weeks old (The Jackson Laboratory, 005557)
- Biosafety hood
- Ketamine/xylazine/saline mixture (20:2.5:77.5, v/v/v)
- Buprenorphine (Buprenex, 0.3 mg/ml)
- 0.9 % sodium chloride (BD Biosciences, 306500)
- Hair remover lotion (Pharmacy store)
- Individually wrapped alcohol wipes/sterile gauze pads/cotton swab/10 % povidone-iodine
- *Sterile surgical instruments*, including micro dissecting scissors 4.5-in. straight sharp (Roboz, RS-5916)/castroviejo micro dissecting spring scissors (Roboz, RS-5658SC)/μ dissecting forceps, serrated, full curve (Roboz, RS-5138)/μ dissecting forceps, straight, fine sharp tips (Roboz, RS-5090)/wound clip applier, 9 mm (Roboz, RS-9260)/wound clips, 9 mm (Roboz, RS-9265)/wound clip remover (Roboz, RS-9263)
- *Sterile tissue culture instruments*, including 100-mm Petri dishes/50-ml conical tubes/2-ml microcentrifuge tubes
- Instruments for mouse identification
- *Freezing instruments*, including freezing medium (90 % FBS/10 % DMSO, chilled)/2 ml cryovials (VWR 89094-806)/slower freezing chamber (Nalgene, 5100-0001)

1.1.2 Surgical Implantation Process

1. Wash the tumor sample with ~30 ml of ice-cold RPMI1640/1 % penicillin-streptomycin.
2. Transfer the tumor specimen into a 100-mm Petri dish, cut off cystic or necrotic part of the tumor, and wash the tumor specimen with ice-cold RPMI1640/1 % penicillin-streptomycin.

3. Cut the tumor specimen into about 2×2×2 mm fragments, and then wash the tumor pieces gently with ice-cold RPMI1640/1 % penicillin-streptomycin.

4. Optional; place a 2-ml microcentrifuge tube in ice, add 1-ml matrigel, and then further add the cut-small tumor pieces into the tube (make sure all tumor pieces are covered by matrigel) for minimum of 10 min.

5. Weigh a NSG mouse and anesthetize it with ketamine/xylazine/saline mixture (20/2.5/77.5, v/v/v) at 10 μl/g of body weight by intraperitoneal (i.p.) injection.

6. Dilute buprenorphine 1:10 in sterile saline and inject subcutaneously in the loose skin around the neck and shoulder area at 100 μl/mouse.

7. Apply hair remover lotion to the lower back of mice, wait for 15 min, and then wipe the hair off with gauze pads.

8. Wipe the nude skin area with 10 % povidone-iodine followed with sterilization using alcohol wipes.

9. Using surgical scissors, make a 1–1.5 cm vertical incision on the right flank skin, insert straight forceps into the incision up to ~2 cm, and then spread the skin to create a pocket between the skin and the overlying muscle tissue.

10. Using straight forceps, extract a piece of tumor fragment from microcentrifuge tube in which tumor pieces were collected, insert the tumor piece into the incision, and then gently push the tumor further in the pocket. The tumor pieces in this step may be retrieved already coated with matrigel if this was added into the microcentrifuge tube.

11. Close the skin with metallic staples, wipe the incision site with sterile gauze,

12. Repeat steps 7–11 on the left flank skin.

13. Number the mice and then put them back in their cages.

14. Repeat steps 5–13 for more NSG mice. This gives the first cohort F_0.

15. Add the surgery date to your original cage card

16. Check the mice daily and remove wound staples 7-days after surgery.

17. Monitor tumor engraftment (tumor take) and growth weekly, and prepare to passage it into new mice when the tumor reaches ~10 mm in diameter. It may take 1–12 months for primary tissue to engraft and grow in recipient mice.

18. Euthanize tumor-bearing mice, wipe mouse skin over the tumor with alcohol wipes, surgically remove the skin and surrounding interstitial tissue from the tumor, and then remove the tumor mass from the mouse.

19. See step 1–14 to set up the second cohort F_1. Usually 1–3 generations of transplantation may be required to establish a stable mouse line.

20. Flash-freeze several tumor pieces for biological analyses.

21. If there are excess specimens of original tumor or tumor grafts, transfer them into chilled cryovials containing 1.5 ml freezing medium, cap the vials and invert several times, and then place the vials into a slow-freezing chamber such as Mr. Frosty. Immediately place the chamber in a −80 °C freezer for 24 h and then transfer to liquid nitrogen for long-term storage.

1.1.3 Commercial Resources

As the establishment of PDX studies is cumbersome and requires experience in this approach, commercial companies and other contract research organizations which develop and maintain PDX models world-wide are available. Some of these are listed below:

Aveo Oncology http://www.aveooncology.com *(Cambridge, Massachusetts, USA),*
Charles River Laboratories http://www.criver.com *(Wilmington, Massachusetts, USA),*
The Jackson Laboratory https://www.jax.org (Bar Harbor, Maine, USA)
Champions Oncology https://championsoncology.com *(Hackensack, New Jersey, USA),*
GenScript http://www.genscript.com *(Piscataway, New Jersey, USA),*
AJES LifeSciences, LLC http://www.ajeslifesciences.com/ (Stony Brook, NY, USA)
Taconic http://www.taconic.com *(Hudson, New York, USA)*
SAGE Research Labs https://www.horizondiscovery.com (St. Louis, MO, USA)
Crownbio http://www.crownbio.com *(Santa Clara, California, USA),*
Molecular Response Therapeutics http://molecularresponse.com (San Diego, *California, USA)*
Living Tumor Laboratory http://www.livingtumorcentre.com (Vancouver, British Columbia, Canada)
Pharmaron http://www.pharmaron.com (Beijing, China)
WuXi AppTec http://www.wuxiapptec.com (Shanghai, China)
Oncodesign http://www.oncodesign.com (Dijon Cedex, France)
Urolead http://www.urolead.com (Strasbourg, France)
Urosphere http://www.urosphere.com (Toulouse, France)
XenTech http://www.xentech.eu (Paris, France)
Experimental Pharmacology and Oncology http://www.epo-berlin.com (Berlin-Buch, Germany)
Oncotest http://www.oncotest.com (Freiburg, Germany)
Deshpande Laboratories http://www.deshpandelab.com (Bhopal, Madhya Pradesh, India)

1.2 Other Considerations in PDX Models

1.2.1 Cell Lines Versus Intact Tumor Specimen

In vitro-generated human tumor cell lines are often derived from advanced tumors or poorly differentiated neoplasms. Due to the ease of manipulation, cell lines are commonly used for PDX testing platforms in biopharmaceutical companies. However, selective pressure from cell culture often generates tumor cell population likely arising from least differentiated cells. This may result in a loss of important biological properties relative to the parent tumor. Secondly, cell lines have the disadvantage that this selective pressure often results in loss of some clones under the in vitro growth condition. Thus, many cell lines may lose the intra-tumor heterogeneity present in the primary tumor and do not represent the inter-tumor heterogeneity found among different patients. PDX models utilizing whole tumor cell preparation either intact or as cell suspension, however, do maintain the architecture, morphology, and histology of the original tumor, hence are closer to providing a more accurate picture of the primary tumor. This allows in principle for investigating different cancers hence capturing the diversity that exists among different sub-type. Furthermore, the cells have adapted to growth in vitro that is different from the natural tumor environment from which they were derived. Adding to this is the observation that genetic mutations do arise as a result of selective pressure in vitro that are distinct from those seen in the patient [21]. For these reasons, mouse xenograft models of human cell lines often have poor predictive value for translating therapeutics of interest to the clinic. While information garnered from their use can say something about drug efficacy in the immunodeficient mice, in many cases, these models only partially predict efficacy in the clinic and in some cases, the PDX data was largely discordant from the clinical trial built upon them [22]. In this regard, PDX models of intact tumor specimen or tumor cell suspension is superior in terms of recapitulating the growth and histopathological features/characteristics of the original patient tumor.

Because of the homogeneity often associated with the tumor cell population in cell lines, they lack primary host-derived stroma. Primary tumor PDX models, on the other hand, have intact stroma, hence, they are an ideal platform to study tumor–stroma interactions. Furthermore, PDX of primacy tumor sample at least in the initial in vivo passage phase generally bear close resemblance in terms of genetic/genomic landscape and overall physiology when compared with the tumors of patients from which the PDX were derived [3, 19]. In the same vein, histology/morphology [21, 23], transcriptome [22] copy number variations [24], and clonal evolution [25, 26] are often not divergent.

While cell lines, intact tumor tissue or dissociated into cell suspension are the more common forms used for implantation, patient cancer biopsy or specimen can be manipulated in other forms prior to implantation. For example, spheroids have been used in some studies. This is essentially a piece of the tumor tissue that is enzymatically digested and grown in specialized chambers with growth medium prior to implantation. This reduces the vigorous manipulation that is typically associated with single cell suspension preparations [27]. Spheroids retain the histology and genetic pattern of parent tumor and likely preserve the tumor-initiating cells. Another option is to sort (tumor cells) from the disaggregated malignant tissue by FACS based on phenotypic expression of relevant cell surface markers. This approach is particularly useful when studies are focused on understanding contributions of certain sub-populations to tumorigenesis such as cancer stem cells, or metastasis such as tumor-propagating cells, etc.

1.2.2 Heterotopic Versus Orthotopic PDX Models

Orthotopic models are generally considered more accurate in terms of histology and gene expression profile between primary tumor and implanted tumor possibly due to effects of the microenvironment. Heterotopic implantation such as sub-cutaneous route, on the other hand, has been shown to produce tumors with growth properties different from orthotopic models, hence may be divergent from what might be seen in a patient [28, 29]. In this regard, they are thought to be better predictors of patient response to drugs compared to heterotopic implantation models. Most s.c. tumors do not metastasize and may be poor models to study highly aggressive tumors with metastatic potential in humans. As demonstrated by others, most s.c. tumor implantations exhibit a rather benign behavior with growth being confined mostly to the local area of implantation [30]. While metastasis is more permissive in orthotopic models, the form in which the tissue is grafted also impacts level of metastasis. For instance, use of tumors disaggregated into cell suspensions or cell lines often yields low frequencies of metastasis [31]. The downside to orthotopic models is that they are time consuming, and may require imaging techniques to confirm successful implantation as well as tumor growth.

1.3   Humanized PDX Models

Given the lack of an intact immune system in the immuno-deficient recipients mice often used in PDX models, they are not suitable for evaluating stroma–tumor interactions and contribution of immune cells which are now being appreciated as key to shaping the course of tumor growth and progression. To circumvent this challenge, immunodeficient mice such as NOD.SCID mice are now being reconstituted with bone marrow or peripheral blood cells along with the patient tumor implant [32]. This approach allows for generation of what is now termed "humanized" xenograft models. These humanized mice provide a valuable platform for studying how the xenogeneic immune cells recruited to the human tumor contribute to the overall anti-tumor immunity. In addition, immunotherapy drugs aimed at mobilizing the effector arm of the immune system can be studied using these models. A key issue that remains unresolved is to what extent the phenotype and function of the human immune cells transferred into the murine environment recapitulate the response of equivalent cells in their primary human host. One might speculate potential reactivity that are driven by human cells recognizing mouse tissue as foreign (not driven by the tumor milieu) may be erroneously interpreted as anti-tumor response especially with ex-vivo assays that attempt to test effector function of T lymphocytes derived from these models using T cell receptor-independent stimulators such as PMA and Ionomycin. There is also the potential graft versus host disease which may develop over time but this can be largely mitigated by keeping the experimental set up and analysis to a reasonable time frame of 6–10 weeks. As more and more investigators are utilizing this platform as "wholistic" approach to studying tumor biology in concert with associated stroma, efforts are underway to improve these models and apply them to various human cancer types. Currently, there are a number of humanized models mostly for hematologic malignancies such as lymphoblastic leukemia and acute myeloid leukemia [33].

1.4   History of PDX Models

The first PDX was performed by Rygaard and Povlsen when they implanted subcutaneously, a colon cancer specimen from a 71-year-old patient into nude mice which lack T cells. The tumor was reported to have grown as several nodules in the implanted area and exhibited a well differentiated adenocarcinoma histology, similar to that of the patient [34]. PDX performed today are not substantially different from that performed by Rygaard and colleagues [34]. PDX models have been under investigation for several decades with improvements with each succeeding decade. Some of these improvements come from the recipient mice used for the human tissue grafting. Although the use of athymic nude mice has been widespread, newer and more stringent immuno-deficient mice such as NOD.SCID and NOG/NSG mice are gaining traction in their utility especially in experimental settings involving co-implantation of tumor and other cell types.

In a seminal study, Wang and Sordat injected colon cancer cell suspensions into the descending region of the large intestine of nude mice. In this study, local tumor growth as well as metastasis was observed [29]. This was among the first cases of orthotopic implantation as opposed to heterotopic. Hoffman and colleagues were (also) among the pioneers of the orthotopic implantation of intact tumor tissue [35]. Their colon cancer orthotopic PDX model demonstrated robust tumor growth and metastasis. Since then, myriads of various PDX have been conducted in colon, pancreatic, breast, ovarian, lung, head and neck, and stomach cancers [28, 35–40]. The metastatic behavior of these orthotopic tumor grafts seems to be highly concordant with metastatic lesions that developed in patients [28]. In the case of stomach cancer, the primary tumor spread to the peritoneal region and the liver in some patients, an observation that was reproduced when the tumor tissue was placed in mice in PDX studies [28]. Similarly, PDX model of HER2+ cervical cancer was described by Hoffman and colleagues with multi-tissue invasion including lung, liver, peritoneal, and lymph node metastasis in nude mice which reflected the pattern associated with the patient's tumor [32]. Lastly, the efforts of Fidler and co. is thought to be among several key ones that brought some spotlight and interest in the orthotopic tumor models [31].

1.5   Importance of PDX Models

Animal models are invaluable tools for evaluating efficacy, potential toxicity, and side effects of drugs before considering applicability to clinic. PDX models are well suited for this purpose providing an investigational platform to study tumor biology with pre-clinical and translational relevance. Because of their close recapitulation of primary tumors, they allow for investigating tumor biology including cell differentiation, cell death, morphology, architecture, genotype, phenotype, cellular and molecular features associated with tumor growth. As for drug screening, PDX models also offers opportunities to identify biomarkers of drug response/sensitivity providing opportunities for identification of new targets. To a limited extent, they are also of value in pharmacokinetic/pharmacodynamic studies, toxicity studies, and establishing or predicting tolerable dose range at which tumor cells might become sensitive to potential anti-cancer drugs. While PDX models are a great tool for oncology research particularly for pre-clinical efficacy studies, they are often cost and labor intensive. (The formation of) consortia such as the Center of Resource for Experimental Models of Cancer (CreMec), the Translational Proof-of-Concept consortia TransPoc) and the Euro PDX consortium have mechanisms in place to facilitate collaborative research built on PDX models and should be instrumental in making these models of wider application in oncology at reasonable costs.

2   PDX in Various Cancer Types

2.1   Colorectal Cancer

Several investigators have utilized PDX models as platforms to study molecular and genotypic features of colorectal cancer (CRC) [41–44]. Propagation of the tumors in vivo has been conducted with as many as 14 passages as tumor engraftment rate is considered good (at least 70 %) in these models [43]. PDX models are also gaining usefulness in uncovering pathways that may contribute to tumor resistance to drugs. In a CRC study, PDX were treated with cetuximab, an EGFR inhibitor. Assessment of mutation status and gene expression profiling was used to predict sensitivity and response to cetuximab. Mutations in KRAS, NRAS, BRAF and activated MET or low EGFR were associated with decreased response. Furthermore, MET activation was considered key mechanism contributing to resistance to cetuximab [45]. In a retrospective study, resistance to cetuximab was predicted based on presence of KRAS, NRAS, BRAF mutations while HER2 amplification appeared to confer resistance in tumors without these mutations demonstrating the utility of PDX models in deciphering molecular mechanisms that may be engaged by tumor cells to circumvent drug efficacy. These studies highlight how data generated from PDX analyses could inform design of treatment regimen to complement or replace existing ones for effective management of cancer sub-types in which such mechanisms are dominant. As data emerge demonstrating that refractoriness to certain drugs may be in part due to tumor-initiating cancer stem cells, evaluating their distribution within tumors could shed some light on how well as particular sub-type might respond to therapy. Indeed, PDX using patient colorectal cancer tissue was utilized in this context to describe a subset of cancer stem cells [46].

2.2 Pancreatic Cancer

In pancreatic cancer, both cell lines and patient tumor tissue have been used as xenografts. Heavy desmoplasia is a common feature in prostate cancer and one that has implications for drug pharmacokinetics. As cell lines PDX may have less associated stroma compared to whole tissue grafts, results of drug efficacy studies need to be interpreted with caution as they may not mirror drug penetrance in whole tumor xenograft which is often associated with heavy stroma arising from desmoplasia. A number of early studies were conducted in an attempt to identify molecular signatures that could serve as predictive biomarkers [47]. In one study, high basal expression of p70 S6 Kinase was identified as a biomarker predictive of patient's response to mTOR inhibitor treatment [48]. The results from patients, however, were not in alignment with this prediction. By using tumor biopsies and ex-vivo assays to screen for drug efficacies, another pancreatic ductal adenocarcinoma PDX study was able to identify cyclin B1 as a biomarker of response associated with tumor cell growth inhibition by a polo-like kinase inhibitor especially in gemcitabine-refractory pancreatic cancer cells [49]. The use of PDX models as surrogates or xenopatients is also another avenue that has been explored in a number of tumor models including pancreatic cancer. Patient tumor sample is propagated in vivo and tested against a panel of promising agents with the aim of finding regimen that will most likely yield objective response in the patient as informed by the xenograft studies. This approach was explored in a patient whose tumor had PALB2 mutation. Information from genomic studies revealed potential agents with demonstrable anti-tumor activity such as to mitomycin C, a cytostatic agent and cisplatin a chemotherapy drug [50, 51].

The rich stroma often associated with in prostate cancer may in lend itself to immunotherapy. Gemcitabine together with nabplaclitaxel synergized to reduce stroma components and increased the intratumoral levels of gemcitabine, leading to tumor growth inhibition [52]. It is tempting to speculate that the anti-tumor effect seen in this study is in part due to gemcitabine's depleting effect of tumor-associated myeloid cells which are often abundantly represented within the tumor microenvironment [53]. Thus, with a reduction in this immune cell population, which incidentally likely includes immune-suppressive cells (MDSCs, [53], adaptive anti-tumor response becomes less obstructed, potentiating the observed anti-tumor response. Although a phase I/II clinical trial based on these studies showed improved median survival in patients with advanced disease, more studies are warranted to better understand how therapeutic agents with potential to disrupt the tumor cellular composition particularly in pancreatic cancer may shape the outcome of a patient's tumor.

2.3   Lung Cancer

Lung cancer remains among the most prevalent types of cancer. While targeted therapies with small molecule inhibitors have yielded some promising results in patients [54], their effect are often short-lived and there is still a need for agents with potential to effect durable response. In this regard, the use of PDX models have been employed in lung cancer settings to identify mechanisms of drug resistance to existing agents such as docetaxel, and cisplatin or identify biomarkers for predicting therapeutic response such as DNA repair pathways [55, 56].

PDX studies are also well documented for lung cancer [56–58]. In one report, patient tumor specimen were implanted under the sub-renal capsule of NOD.SCID mice which yielded '95% engraftment rate. This study demonstrated the closeness of the PDX tumor to parent tumor in terms of genetic abnormalities but acquired mutation that can occur in persistent tumors [57]. One potential application of PDX models in lung cancer is their use to predict disease course. In a study in which surgically resected tumors from NSCLC patients were used to generate PDX, those samples with successful engraftment were associated with squamous histology with poor differentiation and large tumors in patients who had shorter disease-free survival [59]. This study highlights the fact that post engraftment growth features of xenografts could be considered as predictive of growth pattern in patients and potential for relapse in cases where surgery successfully removed most or all tumor nodules.

Current existing methods of gene sequencing allow for identification of mutations in putative oncogenes or tumor suppressor genes that have the potential to activate or inhibit oncogenic pathways, respectively. What is needed is placing some of these genomic alterations in context with immune activation pathways to gain a more comprehensive understanding of how the regulation of these genes impinges on contribution of the immune system to cancer pathogenesis.

2.4   Melanoma

Murine studies of melanoma have historically used cell lines with varying metastatic potential. While PDX models have been explored, interest in their use in melanoma setting has not been on the same level as other cancers such as breast, lung, ovary, and colon cancer. Reasons for this have been obscure. One early study investigated the effect of anti-tumor agents on cell lines derived from a patient's primary melanoma tissue as well as PDX-derived tumor tissue [59]. There were some concordance in the results seen between the two tumor cell sources but differential sensitivities were also noted for some other agents. These studies were conducted in pre-genomics era, otherwise, they would have benefited from this methodology in terms of understanding molecular networks that may be involved in the discordant findings. More recently, melanoma PDX models have been conducted by multiple groups including those demonstrating the presence of melanoma-initiating cells that appear to be crucial for tumor propagation [60] and a uveal melanoma PDX model which while demonstrating sensitivity to temozolomide, a chemotherapy drug, had poor engraftment rate [61].

With the availability of gene arrays, one group reported a gene signature (as identified by DNA array analyses) that could be predictive of response to 11 cytotoxic anti-cancer agents in a melanoma PDX study [62]. Given that melanoma harbors genetic mutational load that is atop of the spectrum when considering several cancer types side by side, and neo antigens encoded by these mutated genes have been shown to be immunogenic [63], perhaps, PDX models are no longer as relevant for drug discovery for this particular indication in which the natural immune system may be potentiated to eliminate the disease as opposed to often toxic chemotherapy drugs. Based on this line of reasoning, genetically engineered mouse models or models of spontaneous autochthonous development of tumors may be more clinically relevant.

With the advent of antibodies against CTLA4 which was approved for late stage metastatic melanoma by the FDA in 2011 and anti-PD1, approved in 2014, which show clinical efficacy in a subset of patients with advanced melanoma, we are seeing a shift in the management of melanoma towards immunotherapy. In this regard, PDX models might be of less appeal to research scientists and PDX models which largely focus on biology of tumor cells often in isolation from immune cells may be relegated to the backstage.

2.5   Head and Neck Cancer

Unlike melanoma, mutational load in head and neck cancer is relatively low with reports demonstrating mutations in a few tumor suppressor genes such as TP53 [64, 65]. With limited treatment options including chemotherapy and antibodies such as cetuximab, there is a need for investigational platforms such as PDX models to identify new drugs for this challenging cancer type. A number of PDX models focusing on head and neck cancer have been carried out over the years [66–70] but their predictive value for clinical outcome have been somewhat poor. This may be in part due to sub-optimal tumor take reported in some of these studies or unknown factors intrinsic to the design of the study. Good engraftment of patient tumor in PDX models can be predictive of "aggressiveness" of a tumor type but such correlation has not been well established in head and neck cancers. With respect to efforts to use PDX models for drug testing and validation, a phase II clinical study was conducted testing cisplatin and diaziquone in addition to other experimental agents [71]. This study demonstrated that cisplatin had little efficacy in inhibiting tumor growth in the PDX model while diaziquone showed robust cytostatic effect. However, these results were discordant to clinical observations. Mutations that have been reported to contribute to resistance to cisplatin include *TP53* and *CCND1* amplification, a gene involved in cell cycle regulation [72]. Consistent with this report, patients with *TP53* mutation had poor prognosis [73–75]. Despite the overall limited efficacy seen with some of these agents, cetuximab remains one of the drugs of choice among targeted therapy drugs. It will be interesting to see whether combining its strong response in a study of head and neck squamous-cell carcinoma (HNSCC) PDX in which 63 % response was seen [45] could be further improved with co-treatment involving an immuno-modulatory agent. In any case, a number of clinical trials are ongoing to bring the use of some of the experimental agents that have been tested in PDX models to the clinic.

2.6   Breast Cancer

Breast cancer PDX models present with unique issues of consideration such as multiple locations for transplantation sites and responsiveness of sub-types to hormones [76]. The murine environment into which they are implanted may affect their growth and behavior. In this regard, building PDX models that span the different sub-types of breast cancer particularly these hormone-driven ones have been somewhat challenging. However, advances in understanding this dependency through molecular pathway methodologies have led to many great PDX studies some of which incorporate hormone supplementation into their PDX platform in an attempt to mimic as closely as possible, the exposure of the tumor cells to these hormones [21, 76–78]. While tumor takes have not been impressively robust in some of these studies, it has allowed for generation of PDX models to study sub-types based on estrogen, progesterone, and HER2-receptor status. These studies have led to data supporting the observation that triple negative (ER-, PR-, and HER2−) breast cancer presents with aggressive growth pattern and metastatic potential in patients. Armed with these observations, PDX models are now continued to be utilized to evaluate potent anti-cancer drugs to target various breast cancer sub-types. While not applicable to every breast cancer sub-type, it is interesting to note that the engraftment rate and growth of triple negative sub-type in PDX models may be useful as prognostics for patients from which they are derived. In this context, knowledge gained from PDX studies evaluating potential therapeutic drugs of interest could inform of aggressive nature of the disease as well as rational treatment options. While not every PDX model has focused on stromal components, existing reports highlight the contributory role of murine stroma/leukocytes to the tumor microenvironment [21] raising the issue of the extent to which the mouse stromal components alter the human tumor mass. As advances in gene expression profiling methodologies continue, we are likely to see a surge in PDX models aimed at identifying mutations contributing to tumorigenesis. One such mutation, the BRCA2 mutation has been described in which gene expression pattern, the basal-like histology, and stroma showed similarity between the patient tumor and the PDX derivative [78]. With the current era where several "omics" approaches are being explored in an attempt to get a global picture of the overall biology of cancer cells, metabolic pathways through metabolomics is also an area of interest that is being pursued by some investigators [79].

2.7   Prostate Cancer

Limited PDX models exist for prostate cancer in part due to the difficulty in establishing prostate cancer cell lines in vitro. A number of studies have produced successful PDX models with diverse focus [80–84]. The site of implantation is particularly important in prostate cancer PDX as demonstrated by studies in which orthotopic implantation was compared to other sites such as sub-renal and sub-cutaneous spaces [83]. Not surprising, the orthotopic route yielded PDX with best engraftment rate, with tumors with well differentiated histology and which maintained expression of prostate antigen and androgen receptor [83]. Other PDX studies conducted have focused on key biological aspects of prostate cancer pathogenesis including but not limited to angiogenesis [80], genetic mutations [82], tumor stem cells [81], and therapeutic intervention via inhibition of hormones [84]. Given the dearth of PDX studies in prostate cancer, more efforts are warranted for this cancer indication.

2.8   Renal Cell Carcinoma

Both primary patient tumor and cell lines have been utilized for PDX studies in renal cell carcinoma (RCC) [81, 83–88]. The latter has been reported to deviate from the parental tumor as acquired mutations are known to develop with the in vitro culture of RCC cells [89]. A number of treatment options exist for RCC including cytokine therapy and chemo/radiotherapy. However, small molecule inhibitors like Sunitinib and sorafenib, both of which are tyrosine kinase inhibitors [90, 91] are being explored. Using a PDX model, sunitinib was evaluated for anti-cancer effect [90]. This study demonstrated some efficacy but was short lived leading the investigators to implicate epithelial-to-mesenchymal transition as mechanism of resistance [90]. The potential utility of anti-angiogenic drugs as therapeutic agents have also been tested in RCC as studies have demonstrated the human vasculature persists with tumors for a period of time post tumor implantation [80, 92]. Interestingly, sorafenib showed efficacy partially attributed to disrupting inhibition of cell cycle and anti-apoptotic proteins including cyclin B1/D1 and survivin [91]. One of the emerging concepts is combinatorial approaches to target multiple biological processes contributing to RCC. In this vein, an RCC PDX study explored the use anti-angiogenic agent with an inhibitor of mTOR and showed pronounced reduction in blood supply to the xenogeneic tumor [93].

2.9   Glioblastoma Multiforme

Mechanisms driving tumor initiation and progression in Glioblatoma multiforme (GM) are beginning to be unraveled through genomic studies [94]. Due to the complexity of the disease, and the technicality of performing grafts in mice, a number of studies have used athymic nude rats for PDX studies of GM. In one study, patient tumor biopsy was first cultured in vitro to form spheroids which were then subsequently implanted into the cranium of the recipient mice [94]. Results from this study demonstrated the suitability of this orthotopic-recipient host combination as a PDX platform for the diseases and showed the clinical relevance as the tumor behavior such as vascularization was similar to that seen in patients [94]. In another study, anti-VEGF treatment, which has anti-angiogenic activity led to reduction of blood supply to the tumor. Although some shrinkage in tumor was noted, the hypoxic environment within the tumor promoted tumor cell invasion that appeared to rely on the PI3K/AKT signaling pathway undermining durable and long-lasting inhibition of tumor growth. Nevertheless, the similarity between the primary patient biopsy and the PDX-derived tumor sample based on genomic analyses and vasculature undoubtedly makes PDX models of GM ideal investigational platforms to evaluate targeted therapies either as monotherapy or in combination with agents that inhibit angiogenesis.

3   Clinical Utility of PDX

3.1   PDX Models as Tools for Understanding Genomic and Protein Expression Profile of Cancers

Some investigators have also focused their attention on the regulation of genes and gene products involved in cancer pathogenesis such as those involved in migration and angiogenesis [95]. In a study involving several PDX tumor models, tissue microarray focusing on a number of genes including VEGF-A, proteinase-activated receptor 1, cathepsin B, integrin β1, and MMP1 among others was conducted. This analysis provided some picture of molecular features employed in metastasis and angiogenesis. In this regard, gene set enrichment analyses of multiple canonical pathways involved in angiogenesis could also be informative in terms of evaluating metastatic ability of the tumor cells. Existing reports from genome-wide studies have demonstrated that PDX models derived from primary patient tumor are more preserved with respect to global gene expression pattern and pathways, and closely mirror that seen in patients [13, 55]. In an NSCLC PDX study of 17 PDX-tumor sample pairs, 10 were found to have correlation co-efficient of '0.9 as determined from hierarchical clustering analyses [55]. Similarly, a pancreatic cancer tumor-PDX pairing study revealed that 10 out of 12 retain the expression levels of mutant KRAS as well as SMAD4 expression [47]. In a comprehensive study comparing primary small cell lung tumor PDX with cell lines derived from them, substantial changes were reported in gene expression pattern such that cell lines that were derived from an initial PDX and later cultured for several months before implantation had as many as 395 genes that were differentially expressed when compared with the founding PDX tumor [13]. Taken together, these reports highlight the notion that gene expression pattern can change considerably in patient tumors when subjected to extensive in vitro manipulations such as generation of cell lines [13] and some of these changes may be irreversible, thus permanently altering the behavior of in vitro-generated PDX tumor models.

3.2 PDX Models as Tools for Predicting Clinical Response

A great percentage of oncology compounds fail to enter the clinic in part due to the low predictability of the pre-clinical pharmacological model used to text their efficacy. Several lines of evidence show that PDX models have better predictive value for clinical outcome compared to cell line-derived xenograft models. Models in which the heterogeneity and hierarchical complexity of tumors, i.e. tumor-initiating cells, tumor-propagating cells/tumor stem cells are preserved are likely to generate information that is relevant to patient tumors. In this context, PDX models particularly those utilizing patient's tumor tissue which have this feature are of value.

Many clinical trials are designed based on findings from pre-clinical PDX studies [16, 96, 97]. A number of these studies demonstrate high potential of PDX models in predicting objective response in patients in the clinic. In a study of 34 cancer patients, the predicted response or resistance rate for chemotherapy drugs including cetuximab using PDX models was remarkably high, and correlated with patient response [97]. In another study in which cetuximab was tested in metastatic colorectal cancer PDX models at clinically relevant doses (CRD), results mirrored what was seen in the clinic [16, 96]. Similarly, PDX models of small cell lung cancer evaluating efficacy of topotecan as monotherapy or in combination with other agents yielded outcomes that were similar to those in phase II clinical trials [98]. In an effort to identify potential treatment regimen for patients with refractory tumors, patient tumor graft studies were conducted with several agents with anti-cancer properties. This study led to identification of treatment plan for 11 of 14 patients which resulted in nearly 90 % clinical objective response [99].

While the studies above provide supporting evidence for the utilization of PDX models as predictive platforms for clinical studies, there exists a number of reports in which discordant results were observed [100, 101]. In a phase II clinical trials testing therapeutic index of an experimental drug brequinar sodium, marginal clinical response of about 5 % was only seen in lung cancer subjects despite a more robust (63–80 %) response rate as predicted by PDX models [100]. This could be attributed to the relatively small number of the PDX tumors used for the study which likely makes predictive power less accurate. The experimental drug Sagopilone was also tested in NSCLC PDX models and while demonstrating a robust 50 % tumor regression in mice [102], its effect in clinical studies was dismal [101]. Another issue is that disease stage may factor into the course of tumor development and progression in PDX models. Early stage tumors may yield discordant results compared with late stage tumors due to differences in growth properties and metastatic potentials. Furthermore, in cases where resected tumors are used for

PDX studies, they may offer little in terms of forecasting how patients might perform under drugs of investigation especially where surgical re-sectioning in itself was therapeutic.

3.3   Using PDX Models Towards Personalized Cancer Care

One of the utilities of PDX models is the potential for testing novel agents with the hope of translating them to patient application especially in settings where patient's tumor is refractory to existing standard of care or therapeutic options and is advanced. To do this, a piece of patient's tumor needs to be obtained. This could be achieved by biopsy or when surgical re-sectioning is being performed. Then follow the basic series of steps involved in setting up a PDX: implant patient tissue in immunodeficient recipient mice, test a number of drugs, identify those with promise, and subsequently test those in the patient. An example of this is a clinical pilot study in pancreatic cancer [103].

PDX models can also be particularly useful in the drug discovery process including target identification, validation, and drug screening. Tumors refractory to treatment can be propagated in mice to better understand mechanisms of drug resistance by profiling such tumors pre-implantation and identifying pathways that have been amplified or altered relative to treatment-naive tumor sample.

With the re-invigoration of interest in the utilization of PDX model came the concept of "avatars". Although largely used to describe patient-derived xenografts that are implanted sub-cutaneously, the consensus is that they offer the potential to test various drugs on a patient's currently un-resolved cancer. In this regard, modifications to improve PDX avatar models include better and more stringent immunodeficient mice models such as NOD.SCID, NOG/NSG mice.

3.4   PDX as Platforms for Biomarker Discovery

PDX models can also allow for identification of novel biomarkers that can be useful in predicting drug sensitivity or resistance. By exploring genetic and molecular feature of the tumor, PDX platforms can reveal patterns associated with objective response or those associated with little to no efficacy. This information is often useful in guiding patient stratification to choose those who are more likely to benefit from a particular regimen or those in which other treatment course may be warranted. In a study that evaluated the activity of cetuximab against a panel of PDX tumors that included colon cancer, it was found that mutations in the KRAS, BRAF, NRAS genes when present was associated with resistance to cetuximab in colon cancer [45]. Other molecular patterns were also identified which led to evaluation of small molecule inhibitor to target some of the dysregulated pathways identified as biomarkers. In a large study of colorectal PDX tumors, KRAS mutations or *HER2* amplification accounted for resistance to cetuximab and these findings were in accordance with response rates noted in the clinic [104, 105]. Similarly, Olaparib, a PARP inhibitor and vemurafenib, a B-Raf inhibitor were tested in clinical trials and showed demonstrable activity in BRCA1/BRCA2 mutant ovarian cancer, and melanoma, respectively [105–107]. These clinical studies resonated with PDX studies [108, 109] demonstrating that PDX models with the employment of genetic screening tools can be effective platform for identification of biomarkers of therapeutic response.

Besides mutational load, expression pattern of genes in primary tumor or PDX-derived tissues as assessed by genomic tools can reveal underlying gene regulatory mechanisms that correlate with sensitivity or resistance to drugs. In one study utilizing PDX of various solid cancers, DNA microanalysis revealed several genes whose differential expression were associated with sensitivity to a number of chemotherapy drugs [110]. The PCR-based method described by Tentler and colleagues [111] is yet another useful tool that could be instrumental in biomarker identification. They have employed this methodology to assess sensitivity or resistance to a number of small molecule inhibitors [55, 112, 113] and biomarkers identified have been employed in some clinical trials. Thus, DNA microarray analysis and deep sequencing of chromosomal segments can aid our efforts in identifying global gene networks or mutations associated with cancer type and its progression. Furthermore, proteomics offers an avenue to dissect expression pattern of aberrantly expressed protein molecules in patient's cancer. By employing these "omics" approaches, multiple pathways enlisted by various cancers which favor growth and survival can be decoded. With the development of biomarkers such as gene mutations, amplifications, post-translational dysregulation, or over expression of protein molecules, drugs could be designed to target those mechanisms employed by the tumor cells to favor growth, survival, and progression.

With the availability of humanized immunodeficient mice, biomarker discovery extending to immunological parameters would be beneficial in terms of understanding the contributory role of tumor expressed markers favoring tumor evasion. Evaluating the expression of inhibitory pathways at the chromosomal level by RT-PCR or at the protein level by FACS or IHC should provide additional opportunities for biomarker discovery. For instance, the expression level of PD-L1 in many solid cancers has been associated with response to immunotherapeutic drugs such as anti-PD-1 antibody [114]. This is one example where comprehensive assessment of suppressive pathways operative on both tumor cells and immune cells could be informative and of substantial predictive value.

4   Challenges in PDX Models

The many challenges that pose barriers to PDX models as "perfect" pre-clinical investigative platform are numerous, some of which have been mentioned briefly in the preceding sections but will be elaborated here.

1. Cell line-derived PDX generally lack heterogeneity resulting from the in vitro selection process of certain clones over others. It is quite common for cultures passaged over many generations to eventually comprise of a near monoclonal tumor cell population. While patient tumor-derived PDX often exhibit clonal diversity similar to the parental tumor, they are also subject to chromosomal changes with extended in vivo passages. Genetic alterations tend arise in grafted tumors probably due to the fact that less differentiated tumors which tend to be the case for early stage cancers are more unstable [115, 116] and the likelihood of development of acquired secondary mutations increases with prolonged passages [47]. Thus, reliable data are best generated at early passage times when architecture, morphology, and histology of the original tumor are still only minimally perturbed.

2. Engraftment rates vary considerably between different models and different cancer types. For example, breast cancer PDX models are generally more challenging compared to other cancers with basal-like cancer models being easier to generate compared to luminal tumors such as the estrogen receptor-positive cancers [18, 76, 77, 103]. The lack of engraftment due to a number of factors including technical failure can also be an impediment to successful PDX model generation. Latency phase is another issue of concern in PDX models. A prolonged latency period [41, 115] before tumor engraftment and growth is confirmed can pose barriers to therapeutic studies in "xenopatient" settings where results are anticipated to guide selection of rational treatment options for aggressive tumor types.

3. Of importance is the stroma or lack thereof surrounding a PDX tumor [117]. Due to the changes in the stroma environment to which the patient tumor is now exposed when present, stromal-associated genes can be dysregulated [19, 116]. Furthermore, the cellular composition of the PDX stroma which may be of human origin initially, eventually becomes replaced with murine equivalent, making inferences about tumor–stroma interactions not so straightforward. Similarly, as with a described renal cell carcinoma model [80, 92], the vasculature of human origin associated with the PDX tumor gradually disappears, paving way for murine vasculature. This is particularly important when considering the impact of soluble factors and angiogenic properties that are important in the biology of a cancer indication. If of mouse origin, they may affect tumor behavior differently than the human equivalents, hence generate outcomes that are divergent from what is seen in a patient. On a related note, PDX models may not faithfully recapitulate their parental counterpart due to differences in hormones present in primary versus secondary host which is relevant for hormone-driven tumors such as sub-types of breast cancer [76, 118–121].

4. While implantation is not particularly difficult, the skills required are notwithstanding beyond that needed for simple maintaining cell cultures in vitro, necessitating an expert in this approach to be a part of the research team. While PDX models are a great tool for oncology research particularly for pre-clinical efficacy studies, they are often cost and labor intensive. Consortia such as the Center of Resource for Experimental Models of Cancer (CreMec), the Translational

Proof-of-Concept consortia TransPoc), and the Euro PDX consortium have mechanisms in place to facilitate collaborative research built on PDX models and should be instrumental in making these models of wider application in oncology at reasonable costs, hence alleviating this potential cost-associated challenge.

5. PDX models might not be very effective in early stage disease as there is about 40–60 % tumor development rate in grafted mice [122] and even then, only malignant, potentially aggressive tumor may effectively engraft and propagate in the recipient mice making PDX model not ideal for early tumors. Additionally, many PDX especially s.c. implants are not metastatic which is a critical determinant in the clinical outcome of disease [30, 31]. This limits the extension of data generated from s.c. PDX systems focused on drug efficacy to human cases especially where such parental tumor has confirmed metastatic potential.

6. Animal use ethical concerns are not to be taken lightly when designing and establishing PDX programs. Many institutions have regulatory committees such as Institutional Review Board (IRB) and Institutional Animal Care and Use Committee (IACUC) that oversee protocols utilized for conducting animal studies and criteria for endpoint assessments including limits of tumor burden allowed in a recipient animal. These regulations ensure smooth operation of animal studies and are not barriers to effectively conducting PDX studies as long as they are abided by.

4.1 Tumor–Host Interactions; Tumor Stroma and Cancer-Associated Cells

The host stromal components and blood vessels contribute to the tumor microenvironment as revealed by studies utilizing secondary recipient transgenic mice expressing fluorescent proteins such as RFP, and GFP [123]. Such studies highlight the contribution of the tumor stroma to tumor progression and behavior in PDX models. The question is: with each passage, does the contribution of the host stroma change enough to alter the behavior of the PDX in a manner that is divergent from the parent tumor? In early stages of PDX implantation, human stroma associated with the tumor is present and has been studied. Both fibroblasts and tumor-infiltrated T cells were readily identified in the implanted PDX tumor of a non-small cell lung cancer model several weeks after implantation [6]. With increasing passaging, stromal components of human origin became replaced with the host (mouse) stroma [76, 78, 123]. Of consideration is the possibility that stroma composition may also impact the pharmacology (pharmacokinetics) of therapeutic agents. In a study evaluating the efficacy of gemcitabine and nab-paclitaxcel in pancreatic PDX tumors, the combination of the drug interestingly was associated with near 3-fold increase in the levels of gemcitabine present in the tumor [124]. Given the potential for gemcitabine to cause a depletion in myeloid cell subset in tumor-bearing mice [125], such increased penetrance of drug may be attributed to re-shaping of the tumor cellular dynamics. Whether the mouse stroma that eventually envelopes the human PDX makes for easier penetration of therapeutic drugs of interest compared to human stroma remains to be seen.

In some PDX models, lack of intact tumor stroma similar to the patient's may essentially preclude studying interactions between tumor cells and both innate and adaptive immune system which are critical to tumor progression and metastasis. Even when present, studying the cross talk between these immune cells and cancer cells may be challenging as the mouse environment may cause some tumor-resident immune cells not to persist, hence become lost due to absence of key growth/survival factors in the secondary host. With this realization in mind, evaluation of immunotherapeutic compounds which rely on the host's immune cells for anti-tumor therapy may be difficult to achieve in PDX models as recipients (immunode-ficient mice) are generally devoid of an intact immune environment.

5   Pushing PDX Beyond the Status Quo

Genomics and sequencing are often tools employed to identify genetic changes favoring tumor growth. These changes provide the recipe for designing targeted therapies for cancers harboring such genomic alterations. In similar vein, epigenetic modifications deserve our attention even in PDX models as information continue to emerge demonstrating how methylation and acetylation patterns impact gene expression. Lastly, proteomics approach can be relied upon for evaluating expression levels of protein of interest as relevant to specific cancer indications such as receptor tyrosine kinases, hormone receptors, growth factor receptors, inhibitory ligands, etc. PDX models have come a long way but could still benefit from refinements. Incorporating many of these analytical tools in PDX tumors will likely provide researchers a more comprehensive picture of regulatory networks at play in cancer tumorigenesis and pathogenesis as well as clues to how components of these networks might be con-nected and employed by cancer cells to evade drugs or immune recognition.

6   Conclusion

Summarily, PDX models are a useful investigational platform to study the many facets of cancer biology. Importantly, they offer an approach to generate an expan-sive array of various human tumors which is essential in order to capture the hetero-geneity that exists among human cancers both within the same cancer type or between different cancers. They are also a great tool for drug discovery, as well as uncovering mechanisms of resistance and sensitivity to known anti-cancer drugs. PDX models are thus a great pre-clinical model given the information they provide us such as histology, genomic landscape, architecture, growth behavior, genetic and epigenetic features as they relate to the primary patient tumor.

PDX models are also a great alternative to GEMMs as they appear to mimic more closely the overall biological parameters associated with the patient's cancer. Lastly, toxicity and tolerability issues need to be weighed carefully when utilizing PDX models given the difference in the body mass between mice and men to avoid over or understating effects when extending drug efficacy studies from PDX mice to human trials. It would be advantageous if there exists certain ground rules on when the results of a PDX study should be deemed robust enough to extrapolate from it and use findings to guide design of clinical trials. As PDX models continue to be employed in oncology, modifications including adoptive transfer of human cells should provide a more rounded approach to understanding tumor biology. After all, cancer cells are never in isolation and their surrounding stroma which includes immune cells are key to course of disease progression.

References

1. Kopetz S, Lemos R, Powis G (2012) The promise of patient-derived xenografts: the best laid plans of mice and men. Clin Cancer Res 18(19):5160–5162
2. Ruggeri BA, Camp F, Miknyoczki S (2014) Animal models of disease: pre-clinical animal models of cancer and their applications and utility in drug discovery. Biochem Pharmacol 87(1):150–161
3. Tentler JJ et al (2012) Patient-derived tumour xenografts as models for oncology drug development. Nat Rev Clin Oncol 9(6):338–350
4. Morvan MG, Lanier LL (2015) NK cells and cancer: you can teach innate cells new tricks. Nat Rev Cancer 16(1):7–19
5. Ito M et al (2002) NOD/SCID/gamma(c) (null) mouse: an excellent recipient mouse model for engraftment of human cells. Blood 100(9):3175–3182
6. Shultz LD et al (2005) Human lymphoid and myeloid cell development in NOD/LtSz-scid IL2R gamma null mice engrafted with mobilized human hemopoietic stem cells. J Immunol 174(10):6477–6489
7. Quintana E et al (2008) Efficient tumour formation by single human melanoma cells. Nature 456(7222):593–598
8. Simpson-Abelson MR et al (2008) Long-term engraftment and expansion of tumor-derived memory T cells following the implantation of non-disrupted pieces of human lung tumor into NOD-scid IL2Rgamma (null) mice. J Immunol 180(10):7009–7018
9. End DW et al (2001) Characterization of the antitumor effects of the selective farnesyl protein transferase inhibitor R115777 in vivo and in vitro. Cancer Res 61(1):131–137
10. Johnson JI et al (2001) Relationships between drug activity in NCI preclinical in vitro and in vivo models and early clinical trials. Br J Cancer 84(10):1424–1431
11. Voskoglou-Nomikos T, Pater JL, Seymour L (2003) Clinical predictive value of the in vitro cell line, human xenograft, and mouse allograft preclinical cancer models. Clin Cancer Res 9(11):4227–4239
12. Van Cutsem E et al (2004) Phase III trial of gemcitabine plus tipifarnib compared with gemcitabine plus placebo in advanced pancreatic cancer. J Clin Oncol 22(8):1430–1438
13. Daniel VC et al (2009) A primary xenograft model of small-cell lung cancer reveals irreversible changes in gene expression imposed by culture in vitro. Cancer Res 69(8):3364–3373
14. Abaan OD et al (2013) The exomes of the NCI-60 panel: a genomic resource for cancer biology and systems pharmacology. Cancer Res 73(14):4372–4382
15. Williams SA et al (2013) Patient-derived xenografts, the cancer stem cell paradigm, and cancer pathobiology in the 21st century. Lab Invest 93(9):970–982

16. Bertotti A et al (2011) A molecularly annotated platform of patient-derived xenografts ("xenopatients") identifies HER2 as an effective therapeutic target in cetuximab-resistant colorectal cancer. Cancer Discov 1(6):508–523

17. Julien S et al (2012) Characterization of a large panel of patient-derived tumor xenografts representing the clinical heterogeneity of human colorectal cancer. Clin Cancer Res 18(19):5314–5328

18. Petrillo LA et al (2012) Xenografts faithfully recapitulate breast cancer-specific gene expression patterns of parent primary breast tumors. Breast Cancer Res Treat 135(3):913–922

19. Reyal F et al (2012) Molecular profiling of patient-derived breast cancer xenografts. Breast Cancer Res 14(1):R11

20. Mattie M et al (2013) Molecular characterization of patient-derived human pancreatic tumor xenograft models for preclinical and translational development of cancer therapeutics. Neoplasia 15(10):1138–1150

21. DeRose YS et al (2011) Tumor grafts derived from women with breast cancer authentically reflect tumor pathology, growth, metastasis and disease outcomes. Nat Med 17(11):1514–1520

22. Zhao X et al (2012) Global gene expression profiling confirms the molecular fidelity of primary tumor-based orthotopic xenograft mouse models of medulloblastoma. Neuro Oncol 14(5):574–583

23. Loukopoulos P et al (2004) Orthotopic transplantation models of pancreatic adenocarcinoma derived from cell lines and primary tumors and displaying varying metastatic activity. Pancreas 29(3):193–203

24. Morton CL, Houghton PJ (2007) Establishment of human tumor xenografts in immunodeficient mice. Nat Protoc 2(2):247–250

25. Ding L et al (2013) Advances for studying clonal evolution in cancer. Cancer Lett 340(2):212–219

26. Gerlinger M et al (2012) Intratumor heterogeneity and branched evolution revealed by multiregion sequencing. N Engl J Med 366(10):883–892

27. Chin L, Andersen JN, Futreal PA (2011) Cancer genomics: from discovery science to personalized medicine. Nat Med 17(3):297–303

28. Furukawa T et al (1993) Nude mouse metastatic models of human stomach cancer constructed using orthotopic implantation of histologically intact tissue. Cancer Res 53(5):1204–1208

29. Wang WR, Sordat B, Piguet D, Sordat M (1982) Human colon tumors in nude mice: implantation site and expression of the invasive phenotype. In: Sordat B (ed) Immune-deficient animals—4th international workshop on immune-deficient animals in experimental research, Karger, Basel, Switzerland. pp 239–245

30. Garralda E et al (2014) Integrated next-generation sequencing and avatar mouse models for personalized cancer treatment. Clin Cancer Res 20(9):2476–2484

31. Fidler IJ (1990) Critical factors in the biology of human cancer metastasis: twenty-eighth G.H.A. Clowes memorial award lecture. Cancer Res 50(19):6130–6138

32. Hiroshima Y et al (2015) Establishment of a patient-derived orthotopic Xenograft (PDOX) model of HER-2-positive cervical cancer expressing the clinical metastatic pattern. PLoS One 10(2):e0117417

33. Meyer LH, Debatin KM (2011) Diversity of human leukemia xenograft mouse models: implications for disease biology. Cancer Res 71(23):7141–7144

34. Rygaard J, Povlsen CO (1969) Heterotransplantation of a human malignant tumour to "Nude" mice. Acta Pathol Microbiol Scand 77(4):758–760

35. Fu XY et al (1991) Models of human metastatic colon cancer in nude mice orthotopically constructed by using histologically intact patient specimens. Proc Natl Acad Sci U S A 88(20):9345–9349

36. Astoul P et al (1996) A patient-like human malignant pleural mesothelioma nude-mouse model. Oncol Rep 3(3):483–487

37. Fu X, Guadagni F, Hoffman RM (1992) A metastatic nude-mouse model of human pancreatic cancer constructed orthotopically with histologically intact patient specimens. Proc Natl Acad Sci U S A 89(12):5645–5649

38. Fu X, Hoffman RM (1993) Human ovarian carcinoma metastatic models constructed in nude mice by orthotopic transplantation of histologically-intact patient specimens. Anticancer Res 13(2):283–286
39. Fu X, Le P, Hoffman RM (1993) A metastatic orthotopic-transplant nude-mouse model of human patient breast cancer. Anticancer Res 13(4):901–904
40. Wang X, Fu X, Hoffman RM (1992) A new patient-like metastatic model of human lung cancer constructed orthotopically with intact tissue via thoracotomy in immunodeficient mice. Int J Cancer 51(6):992–995
41. Dangles-Marie V et al (2007) Establishment of human colon cancer cell lines from fresh tumors versus xenografts: comparison of success rate and cell line features. Cancer Res 67(1):398–407
42. Fichtner I et al (2004) Anticancer drug response and expression of molecular markers in early-passage xenotransplanted colon carcinomas. Eur J Cancer 40(2):298–307
43. Guenot D et al (2006) Primary tumour genetic alterations and intra-tumoral heterogeneity are maintained in xenografts of human colon cancers showing chromosome instability. J Pathol 208(5):643–652
44. Linnebacher M et al (2010) Cryopreservation of human colorectal carcinomas prior to xenografting. BMC Cancer 10:362
45. Krumbach R et al (2011) Primary resistance to cetuximab in a panel of patient-derived tumour xenograft models: activation of MET as one mechanism for drug resistance. Eur J Cancer 47(8):1231–1243
46. Dalerba P et al (2007) Phenotypic characterization of human colorectal cancer stem cells. Proc Natl Acad Sci U S A 104(24):10158–10163
47. Rubio-Viqueira B et al (2006) An in vivo platform for translational drug development in pancreatic cancer. Clin Cancer Res 12(15):4652–4661
48. Garrido-Laguna I et al (2010) Integrated preclinical and clinical development of mTOR inhibitors in pancreatic cancer. Br J Cancer 103(5):649–655
49. Jimeno A et al (2010) A fine-needle aspirate-based vulnerability assay identifies polo-like kinase 1 as a mediator of gemcitabine resistance in pancreatic cancer. Mol Cancer Ther 9(2):311–318
50. Jones S et al (2009) Exomic sequencing identifies PALB2 as a pancreatic cancer susceptibility gene. Science 324(5924):217
51. Villarroel MC et al (2011) Personalizing cancer treatment in the age of global genomic analyses: PALB2 gene mutations and the response to DNA damaging agents in pancreatic cancer. Mol Cancer Ther 10(1):3–8
52. Von Hoff DD et al (2011) Gemcitabine plus nab-paclitaxel is an active regimen in patients with advanced pancreatic cancer: a phase I/II trial. J Clin Oncol 29(34):4548–4554
53. Talmadge JE, Gabrilovich DI (2013) History of myeloid-derived suppressor cells. Nat Rev Cancer 13(10):739–752
54. Gross S et al (2015) Targeting cancer with kinase inhibitors. J Clin Invest 125(5):1780–1789
55. Fichtner I et al (2008) Establishment of patient-derived non-small cell lung cancer xenografts as models for the identification of predictive biomarkers. Clin Cancer Res 14(20):6456–6468
56. Nemati F et al (2009) Preclinical assessment of cisplatin-based therapy versus docetaxel-based therapy on a panel of human non-small-cell lung cancer xenografts. Anti-cancer Drugs 20(10):932–940
57. Cutz JC et al (2006) Establishment in severe combined immunodeficiency mice of subrenal capsule xenografts and transplantable tumor lines from a variety of primary human lung cancers: potential models for studying tumor progression-related changes. Clin Cancer Res 12(13):4043–4054
58. Dong X et al (2010) Patient-derived first generation xenografts of non-small cell lung cancers: promising tools for predicting drug responses for personalized chemotherapy. Clin Cancer Res 16(5):1442–1451

59. John T et al (2011) The ability to form primary tumor xenografts is predictive of increased risk of disease recurrence in early-stage non-small cell lung cancer. Clin Cancer Res 17(1):134–141
60. Schatton T et al (2008) Identification of cells initiating human melanomas. Nature 451(7176):345–349
61. Nemati F et al (2010) Establishment and characterization of a panel of human uveal melanoma xenografts derived from primary and/or metastatic tumors. Clin Cancer Res 16(8):2352–2362
62. Fiebig HH et al (2007) Gene signatures developed from patient tumor explants grown in nude mice to predict tumor response to 11 cytotoxic drugs. Cancer Genomics Proteomics 4(3):197–209
63. Rizvi NA et al (2015) Cancer immunology. Mutational landscape determines sensitivity to PD-1 blockade in non-small cell lung cancer. Science 348(6230):124–128
64. Agrawal N et al (2011) Exome sequencing of head and neck squamous cell carcinoma reveals inactivating mutations in NOTCH1. Science 333(6046):1154–1157
65. Stransky N et al (2011) The mutational landscape of head and neck squamous cell carcinoma. Science 333(6046):1157–1160
66. Chen J et al (1996) Xenograft growth and histodifferentiation of squamous cell carcinomas of the pharynx and larynx. Oral Surg Oral Med Oral Pathol Oral Radiol Endod 81(2):197–202
67. Hennessey PT et al (2011) Promoter methylation in head and neck squamous cell carcinoma cell lines is significantly different than methylation in primary tumors and xenografts. PLoS One 6(5):e20584
68. Prince ME et al (2007) Identification of a subpopulation of cells with cancer stem cell properties in head and neck squamous cell carcinoma. Proc Natl Acad Sci U S A 104(3):973–978
69. Wennerberg J, Trope C, Biorklund A (1983) Heterotransplantation of human head and neck tumours into nude mice. Acta Otolaryngol 95(1-2):183–190
70. Zatterstrom UK et al (1992) Growth of xenografted squamous cell carcinoma of the head and neck--possible correlation with patient survival. APMIS 100(11):976–980
71. Langdon SP et al (1994) Preclinical phase II studies in human tumor xenografts: a European multicenter follow-up study. Ann Oncol 5(5):415–422
72. Henriksson E et al (2006) p53 mutation and cyclin D1 amplification correlate with cisplatin sensitivity in xenografted human squamous cell carcinomas from head and neck. Acta Oncol 45(3):300–305
73. Cabelguenne A et al (2000) p53 alterations predict tumor response to neoadjuvant chemotherapy in head and neck squamous cell carcinoma: a prospective series. J Clin Oncol 18(7):1465–1473
74. Koch WM et al (1996) p53 mutation and locoregional treatment failure in head and neck squamous cell carcinoma. J Natl Cancer Inst 88(21):1580–1586
75. Peltonen JK et al (2011) Specific TP53 mutations predict aggressive phenotype in head and neck squamous cell carcinoma: a retrospective archival study. Head Neck Oncol 3:20
76. Marangoni E et al (2007) A new model of patient tumor-derived breast cancer xenografts for preclinical assays. Clin Cancer Res 13(13):3989–3998
77. Beckhove P et al (2003) Efficient engraftment of human primary breast cancer transplants in nonconditioned NOD/Scid mice. Int J Cancer 105(4):444–453
78. de Plater L et al (2010) Establishment and characterisation of a new breast cancer xenograft obtained from a woman carrying a germline BRCA2 mutation. Br J Cancer 103(8):1192–1200
79. Moestue SA et al (2010) Distinct choline metabolic profiles are associated with differences in gene expression for basal-like and luminal-like breast cancer xenograft models. BMC Cancer 10:433
80. Gray DR et al (2004) Short-term human prostate primary xenografts: an in vivo model of human prostate cancer vasculature and angiogenesis. Cancer Res 64(5):1712–1721
81. Grisanzio C et al (2011) Orthotopic xenografts of RCC retain histological, immunophenotypic and genetic features of tumours in patients. J Pathol 225(2):212–221

82. Laitinen S et al (2002) Chromosomal aberrations in prostate cancer xenografts detected by comparative genomic hybridization. Genes Chromosomes Cancer 35(1):66–73
83. Wang Y et al (2005) Development and characterization of efficient xenograft models for benign and malignant human prostate tissue. Prostate 64(2):149–159
84. Yoshida T et al (2005) Antiandrogen bicalutamide promotes tumor growth in a novel androgen-dependent prostate cancer xenograft model derived from a bicalutamide-treated patient. Cancer Res 65(21):9611–9616
85. Angevin E et al (1999) Human renal cell carcinoma xenografts in SCID mice: tumorigenicity correlates with a poor clinical prognosis. Lab Invest 79(7):879–888
86. Beniers AJ et al (1992) Establishment and characterization of five new human renal tumor xenografts. Am J Pathol 140(2):483–495
87. Coppin C et al (2011) Targeted therapy for advanced renal cell cancer (RCC): a Cochrane systematic review of published randomised trials. BJU Int 108(10):1556–1563
88. Kopper L et al (1984) Renal cell carcinoma--xenotransplantation into immuno-suppressed mice. Oncology 41(1):19–24
89. Beroukhim R et al (2009) Patterns of gene expression and copy-number alterations in von-hippel lindau disease-associated and sporadic clear cell carcinoma of the kidney. Cancer Res 69(11):4674–4681
90. Hammers HJ et al (2010) Reversible epithelial to mesenchymal transition and acquired resistance to sunitinib in patients with renal cell carcinoma: evidence from a xenograft study. Mol Cancer Ther 9(6):1525–1535
91. Yuen JS et al (2011) Inhibition of angiogenic and non-angiogenic targets by sorafenib in renal cell carcinoma (RCC) in a RCC xenograft model. Br J Cancer 104(6):941–947
92. Sanz L et al (2009) Differential transplantability of human endothelial cells in colorectal cancer and renal cell carcinoma primary xenografts. Lab Invest 89(1):91–97
93. Ellis L et al (2012) Vascular disruption in combination with mTOR inhibition in renal cell carcinoma. Mol Cancer Ther 11(2):383–392
94. Wang J et al (2009) A reproducible brain tumour model established from human glioblastoma biopsies. BMC Cancer 9:465
95. Smith V et al (2008) Tissue microarrays of human tumor xenografts: characterization of proteins involved in migration and angiogenesis for applications in the development of targeted anticancer agents. Cancer Genomics Proteomics 5(5):263–273
96. Cunningham D et al (2004) Cetuximab monotherapy and cetuximab plus irinotecan in irinotecan-refractory metastatic colorectal cancer. N Engl J Med 351(4):337–345
97. Fiebig HHD, Dengler WA, Roth T (1999) Human tumor xenografts: predictivity, characterization and discovery of new anticancer agents. In: FHHaBAM (eds) Relevance of tumor models for anticancer drug development, Karger, Basel, Switzerland. pp 29–50
98. Nemati F et al (2010) Clinical relevance of human cancer xenografts as a tool for preclinical assessment: example of in-vivo evaluation of topotecan-based chemotherapy in a panel of human small-cell lung cancer xenografts. Anticancer Drugs 21(1):25–32
99. Hidalgo M et al (2011) A pilot clinical study of treatment guided by personalized tumorgrafts in patients with advanced cancer. Mol Cancer Ther 10(8):1311–1316
100. Boven E et al (1992) Phase II preclinical drug screening in human tumor xenografts: a first European multicenter collaborative study. Cancer Res 52(21):5940–5947
101. Heigener DF et al (2013) Prospective, multicenter, randomized, independent-group, open-label phase II study to investigate the efficacy and safety of three regimens with two doses of sagopilone as second-line therapy in patients with stage IIIB or IV non-small-cell lung cancer. Lung Cancer 80(3):319–325
102. Hammer S et al (2010) Comparative profiling of the novel epothilone, sagopilone, in xenografts derived from primary non-small cell lung cancer. Clin Cancer Res 16(5):1452–1465
103. Cottu P et al (2012) Modeling of response to endocrine therapy in a panel of human luminal breast cancer xenografts. Breast Cancer Res Treat 133(2):595–606

104. Amado RG et al (2008) Wild-type KRAS is required for panitumumab efficacy in patients with metastatic colorectal cancer. J Clin Oncol 26(10):1626–1634
105. Karapetis CS et al (2008) K-ras mutations and benefit from cetuximab in advanced colorectal cancer. N Engl J Med 359(17):1757–1765
106. Das Thakur M et al (2013) Modelling vemurafenib resistance in melanoma reveals a strategy to forestall drug resistance. Nature 494(7436):251–255
107. Gelmon KA et al (2011) Olaparib in patients with recurrent high-grade serous or poorly differentiated ovarian carcinoma or triple-negative breast cancer: a phase 2, multicentre, open-label, non-randomised study. Lancet Oncol 12(9):852–861
108. Kortmann U et al (2011) Tumor growth inhibition by olaparib in BRCA2 germline-mutated patient-derived ovarian cancer tissue xenografts. Clin Cancer Res 17(4):783–791
109. Scott CL et al (2013) Patient-derived xenograft models to improve targeted therapy in epithelial ovarian cancer treatment. Front Oncol 3:295
110. Gerber HP, Ferrara N (2005) Pharmacology and pharmacodynamics of bevacizumab as monotherapy or in combination with cytotoxic therapy in preclinical studies. Cancer Res 65(3):671–680
111. Bergers G et al (1999) Effects of angiogenesis inhibitors on multistage carcinogenesis in mice. Science 284(5415):808–812
112. Arbuck SG (1989) Overview of clinical trials using 5-fluorouracil and leucovorin for the treatment of colorectal cancer. Cancer 63(6 Suppl):1036–1044
113. Houghton PJ, Houghton JA (1978) Evaluation of single-agent therapy in human colorectal tumour xenografts. Br J Cancer 37(5):833–840
114. Remon J, Chaput N, Planchard D (2016) Predictive biomarkers for programmed death-1/programmed death ligand immune checkpoint inhibitors in nonsmall cell lung cancer. Curr Opin Oncol 28(2):122–129
115. Bergamaschi A et al (2009) Molecular profiling and characterization of luminal-like and basal-like in vivo breast cancer xenograft models. Mol Oncol 3(5-6):469–482
116. Ding L et al (2010) Genome remodelling in a basal-like breast cancer metastasis and xenograft. Nature 464(7291):999–1005
117. Bhowmick NA, Neilson EG, Moses HL (2004) Stromal fibroblasts in cancer initiation and progression. Nature 432(7015):332–337
118. Clarke R (1996) Animal models of breast cancer: their diversity and role in biomedical research. Breast Cancer Res Treat 39(1):1–6
119. Fingert HJ et al (1987) Rapid growth of human cancer cells in a mouse model with fibrin clot subrenal capsule assay. Cancer Res 47(14):3824–3829
120. Hoehn W et al (1980) Human prostatic adenocarcinoma: some characteristics of a serially transplantable line in nude mice (PC 82). Prostate 1(1):95–104
121. Visonneau S et al (1998) Growth characteristics and metastatic properties of human breast cancer xenografts in immunodeficient mice. Am J Pathol 152(5):1299–1311
122. Jin K et al (2010) Patient-derived human tumour tissue xenografts in immunodeficient mice: a systematic review. Clin Transl Oncol 12(7):473–480
123. Suetsugu A et al (2012) Multi-color palette of fluorescent proteins for imaging the tumor microenvironment of orthotopic tumorgraft mouse models of clinical pancreatic cancer specimens. J Cell Biochem 113(7):2290–2295
124. Von Hoff DD et al (2013) Increased survival in pancreatic cancer with nab-paclitaxel plus gemcitabine. N Engl J Med 369(18):1691–1703
125. Suzuki E et al (2005) Gemcitabine selectively eliminates splenic Gr-1+/CD11b+myeloid suppressor cells in tumor-bearing animals and enhances antitumor immune activity. Clin Cancer Res 11(18):6713–6721

Organoid Culture: Applications in Development and Cancer

Israel Cañadas and David A. Barbie

1 History

The culture of primary human tissues ex vivo has historically been laden with challenges. Following the successful establishment of multiple different carcinoma cell lines, most notably HeLa cells, which helped support viral research in the 1940s and 1950s, the difficulty of propagating normal diploid cells was recognized by multiple investigators. Despite using similar 2-dimensional (2D) culture techniques that have stood the test of time - adherent culture on petri dishes using Eagle's Medium with balanced salt solutions, 10 % calf serum, and penicillin/streptomycin - Hayflick and Moorhead perhaps best defined the limits of studying normal human tissue in a dish in 1961 [1]. Upon mincing fetal tissue they could derive multiple human diploid fibroblast cultures, but invariably the number of subcultivations was limited below 60 passages, for which they coined the term cellular "senescence," also commonly known as the "Hayflick Limit."

It was not until the late 1990s that the discovery of telomerase and the cloning of the human catalytic subunit (hTERT) enabled the immortalization of human diploid fibroblasts, proving a direct association between this limit and telomere dysfunction [2]. Even so, the immortalization of epithelial cells in 2D required also required the inactivation of the pRB/p16 cell cycle checkpoint [3], and growth in 3-dimensions (3D) via cellular transformation necessitated the abrogation of multiple checkpoints by viral oncoproteins and expression of oncogenic RAS [4]. However, shortly following the discovery of hTERT, it was also recognized that its expression was not only observed in germ cell tissues and tumors, but also in certain stem cell compartments such as colonic epithelial crypts [5]. Given their self-renewing potential, it is intuitive that a mechanism to maintain telomere length would be advantageous in

I. Cañadas • D.A. Barbie (✉)
Department of Medical Oncology, Dana Farber Cancer Institute,
450 Brookline Avenue, Boston, MA 02215, USA
e-mail: dbarbie@partners.org

© Springer International Publishing Switzerland 2017   41
A.R. Aref, D. Barbie (eds.), *Ex Vivo Engineering of the Tumor Microenvironment*,
Cancer Drug Discovery and Development, DOI 10.1007/978-3-319-45397-2_3

this setting, but it would take the later isolation of intestinal stem cells to enable direct confirmation of their elevated telomerase activity and downregulation upon differentiation [6]. Thus, the ability to expand normal human tissue ex vivo, let alone organoid structures, seemed like a distant reality even at the turn of the millenium.

Ultimately in the late 2000s it was the seminal work in the study of intestinal crypt biology by the laboratory of Hans Clevers in the Netherlands, coupled with pioneering studies in neurogenesis by Yoshiki Sasai's group in Japan, that provided the blueprint for how to cultivate organoids ex vivo. What follows are detailed descriptions of these discoveries, since they have spawned the emerging field of organoid biology, with broad implications for the study of normal human development and cancer.

Following up on their observation that inactivation of Wnt signaling depleted the intestinal epithelial stem cell compartment in mice [7], the Clevers group set out to identify specific Wnt regulated factors that might mark the stem cell compartment in the small intestine and colon. By systematically analyzing the expression of nearly 80 Wnt target genes, they honed in on *Lgr5* as being uniquely expressed in crypt base columnar cells [8]. Remarkably, using lineage tracing from an *Lgr5* reporter strain in mice, they could show that this specific crypt cell could produce all intestinal epithelial lineages, confirming its role as a true intestinal stem cell. Because of this remarkable potential in vivo, the Clevers laboratory also considered whether these Lgr5+ stem cells could be coaxed into forming such crypt-villus structures in vitro, even in the absence of the native mesenchymal environment [9]. For their 3D culture system the considered the requirement of 4 different factors that they hypothesized as necessary to enable organoid formation: (1) A laminin rich Matrigel to provide architectural support, (2) The Wnt agonist R-spondin 1 to drive important developmental Wnt signaling, (3) Epidermal growth factor (Egf) to provide a known intestinal cell proliferative signal, and (4) Noggin, a bone morphogenetic protein (BMP) antagonist that induces crypt expansion and is also used to help maintain human embryonic stem (ES) or induced pluripotent stem (IPS) cells in an undifferentiated state. Remarkably, these conditions enabled the ex vivo expansion of these Lgr5+ stem cells into crypts that budded and ultimately formed an organoid structure with a central lumen lined by a villus-like epithelium (Fig. 1—reprint with permission). Furthermore, they could be propagated by mechanical dissociation and replanting, with long term culture possible for more than 8 months, and retention of gene expression profiles that matched freshly isolated intestinal crypts, without induction of stress-related genes. Additionally, detailed structural analysis of established organoids revealed the presence of enterocytes with mature brush borders, goblet cells, Paneth cells, and enteroendocrine cells, demonstrating the ability of this system to recapitulate gut physiology in a dish. Thus, identification of the key resident stem cell, coupled with growth conditions supporting the endogenous developmental program, unleashed the potential to culture organoids from a variety of tissues ex vivo.

Around the same time, Yoshiki Sasai's laboratory in Japan was experimenting with strategies in which to recapitulate neurogenesis from mouse ES cells in cell culture. Previously, they had developed a technique using serum free culture of

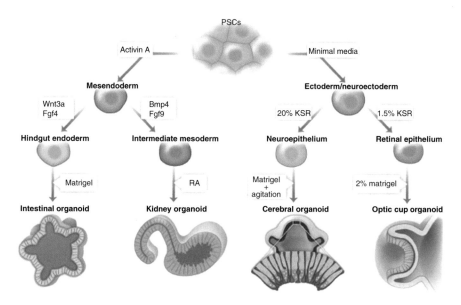

Fig. 1 Schematic representation of organoid differentiation strategies developed from human PSCs. PSCs can be derived into the different germ layers *in vitro* with the indicated differentiation protocols. After the initial germ layer specification, cells are transferred into 3D systems and generate organoids that recapitulate *ex vivo* the developmental steps that occur *in vivo*

embryoid-body like aggregates (SFEB) in suspension, and could demonstrate differentiation into telencephalic progenitors (Bf1/FoxG1+), though at a frequency of less than 50 %[10]. They therefore set out to develop culture conditions in which to improve both the efficiency and differentiation capacity of these cells. By concentrating dissociated ES cells in a low cell-adhesion 96-well plate they could induce "quick" re-aggregation (SFEBq), which not only improved the efficiency of Bf1+ progenitor generation up to 75 %, but also enhanced their differentiation [11]. Remarkably, longer-term culture of these SFEBq aggregates resulted in organization into a neuroepithelial sheet with a polarity similar to the known embryonic structure, and dissociation at day 12 resulted in differentiation of neural progenitors into postmitotic neurons. These neurons could integrate into cortical tissues, and showed spontaneous Ca2+ oscillations over several millimeters, revealing their physiologic potential. Even more impressively, by modifying developmental cues through various supplementation with factors regulating Fgf, Wnt, and BMP signaling they could generate higher order structures ex vivo that recapitulated corticogenesis. Subsequent work from their group expanded the potential of 3D neuronal organoid culture, even demonstrating that the retinal primorium or optic cup could be generated via an intrinsic self-organizing program [12]. Together with the work from the Clevers group, these findings firmly established the ability to culture and engineer organoid structures with remarkable complexity. Below we discuss how these discoveries have currently impacted studies on mouse and human differentiation and development, followed by their application to cell differentiation gone awry, in tumorigenesis.

2   Study of Development

Based upon this foundational work, in vitro 3D organoid cultures have emerged as useful systems to study tissue development, organogenesis and stem cell behavior ex vivo. Indeed, when grown in a 3D environment and in the presence of specific combinations of niche factors, pluripotent stem cells (PSCs) or isolated organ progenitors from a variety of different tissue types have the ability to differentiate and self-assemble to form the cellular organization of the organ itself [9, 13, 14]. Thus, organoids represent a convenient model system with the potential to study development and increase our understanding of how mammals develop from a single toti-potent cell to a complex adult organism. These organoid cultures provide the opportunity to explore human development in a context very similar to development in vivo, and, based upon their ability to recapitulate normal physiology, to study adult homeostasis.

Organoid technologies include exogenous tissue patterning using combination of growth factors that drive particular cell identities and extracellular matrix gel embedding, followed by a reaggregation to stimulate cell movement and create self-organized 3D tissue. By using this culture system as a model for studying organ development, organoids derived from PSCs have been established for gut, liver, kidney, brain and retina, among others (Fig. 1—reprint with permission). For example, organoids for the gastrointestinal (GI) tract and retinal organoids have been used to study comparative human and rodent tissue morphogenesis [15, 16], and brain organoids have been used to evaluate the division of human neural stem cells [17]. Below we detail several examples of how organoid culture has yielded important insights into normal development of different organ types.

2.1   Intestinal Organoids

Several laboratories have generated intestinal organoids from PSCs of mouse or human origin with an architecture and cellular composition remarkably similar to the organ in vivo. In addition, these gut organoids displayed intestinal functions such as absorptive and secretory activity.

As discussed above, the laboratory of Hans Clevers first showed that adult intestinal Lgr5-expressing stem cells could form organoids when cultured in 3D in a laminin-rich Matrigel. These organoids self-organized to form the crypt-villus structures and all major cell-types that constitute the intestine in vivo [9]. These adult-derived mouse organoids could even be transplanted into damaged mouse colon to reconstitute a single-layered epithelium with self-renewing crypts that were functionally and histologically normal [18]. In addition, this system facilitated the identification of Paneth cells as a key component of the crypt niche that supports LGR5 cell development, and, as discussed in detail below, enabled long term culture of dysplastic epithelium from the colon and Barrett's esophagus [19, 20].

Similar principles have also been applied to generate gut organoids from PSCs of human origin as a model for studying human intestinal development. For example, human PSCs can be differentiated in vitro and form organoids with a very similar architecture to the fetal intestine [21]. More recently, an in vivo model of the human small intestine has been developed using pluripotent stem cells, further enabling the study intestinal physiology and disease [22]. Similarly, for the upper gastrointestinal tract, human gastric organoids have been developed that resemble the human stomach through directed in vitro differentiation of human embryonic stem cells and PSCs [23]. Together, these studies describe robust in vitro systems to study the mechanisms underlying human GI development.

2.2 Liver Organoids

Even before the development of these more sophisticated organoid culture techniques, early developmental studies showed that dissociated chick embryonic hepatic tissue can reaggregate and organize into secretory units typical of the liver and consistent with the formation of functional bile ducts [24]. Moreover, recent advances showed that an Lgr5+ progenitor population in the adult mouse liver could form 3D liver organoids when grown in Matrigel. These liver organoids could also be differentiated in vitro to generate functional hepatocytes and transplanted into a mice model of liver disease to partially rescue mortality [25, 26]. A different approach was recently established starting with human PSCs and generating tissues reminiscent of human liver buds [27]. In this case three cell populations were mixed in Matrigel (human PSC-derived hepatic cells, human mesenchymal stem cells and human endothelial cells) to reproduce the early cell lineages of the developing liver. This mixed-cell population generated 3D liver buds that could be ectopically transplanted into mice and performed liver-specific functions. In addition, transplanting human liver buds improved survival in mice subjected to liver injury. Together, these models not only hold promise for further study of hepatogenesis, but may also have future applications in liver transplantation.

2.3 Kidney Organoids

Early reaggregation experiments demonstrated evidence that kidney tissue was capable of self-organization, showing various segments of the nephron and developing the stereotypic organization of the kidney [24, 28]. Recent methodologies used combinations of growth factors to induce renal differentiation. Specifically, culture of kidney PSCs in defined conditions can induce self-organization and generate 3D renal tissues. For example, the exposition of human PSCs to Bmp4 and Fgf2 generated ureteric bud identities, followed by application of retinoic acid, Bmp2 and activin A. To allow further maturation, differentiated cells were co-cultured with mouse embryonic kidney cells to form 3D chimeric organoids [29]. Another study showed that the sequential application of activin A followed by Bmp4 and the Wnt agonist to mouse and human PSCs induced posterior mesoderm differentiation. The application of retinoic acid followed by Fgf9 stimulated cells to assume a meta-nephric mesenchyme identity. By coculturing with embryonic spinal cord, this tissue could produce well-organized nephric tubules and glomerular-like structures [30]. Similarly, stimulation of embryonic stem cells with activin A and Bmp4 generated primitive streak identity. Upon exposure to Fgf9 these cells acquired an intermediate mesoderm identity and spontaneously developed further into ureteric bud and metanephric mesenchyme in the absence of other growth factors. Of note, reaggregation experiments with these cells in 3D allowed more complex tissues generating small, self-organized kidney organoids [31]. Similar to hepatic organoids, the development of these technologies to regenerate the human kidney ex vivo holds future promise for treatment of end stage renal disease.

2.4   Brain Organoids

There is an increasing knowledge about the generation of brain organoids in vitro to study the development of this highly complex organ. Even prior to the work of Sasai, pioneering reaggregation studies using chick neural progenitors demonstrated the intrinsic self-organizing capacity of this organ [32]. Several other studies also used multipotent neural stem cells (NSCs) from PSCs or isolated neuroepithelium to study in vitro neural differentiation; however, because these studies used 2D methodologies, they had many limitations modeling the overall organization of the brain [33]. For this reason, the aforementioned work using alternative 3D culture methods to recapitulate brain tissue organization has been instrumental in demonstrating that particular brain region identities can be generated and self-organize with axial polarity, even from human ES cells [34]. Other regions can also be generated when maintaining cells with specific growth factors. For example, Hedgehog signaling derived ventral forebrain tissue and either Bmp4 and Wnt3a stimulation generated granule neurons [35, 36]. Recently, researchers have also established a method to develop different brain regions in the same organoid. In this case embryoid bodies were embedded in Matrigel, promoting outgrowth of large buds of neuroepithelium, which then expanded and developed into various brain regions, leading to the term "mini-brains"[17]. Thus, brain organoids represent a powerful tool to perform functional studies and to clarify developmental pathways of perhaps the most complicated of all organs.

2.5   Retinal Organoids

The vertebrate retina has represented one of the most powerful reaggregation models in tissue engineering studies for investigating the basis of neural layer development [37]. As discussed above, the advent of brain organoid culture techniques by the Sasai laboratory was extended to the retinal epithelium, which could be generated by using EB aggregates from mouse embryonic stem cells cultured in Matrigel with low serum media [12]. Under these conditions, aggregates spontaneously formed buds of retinal primordial tissue similar to the optic vesicle. These retinal organoids mimicked early retina, displaying markers of neural retina and retinal-pigmented epithelium, retinal stratification with proper apical-basal polarity and morphological tissue shape changes that mimic the stepwise evagination and invagination of the optic cup in vivo. Interestingly, optic cup organoids have also been generated from human PSCs, characterized by some differences when compared to the mouse retina, such as the larger size and the presence of apical nuclear positioning [16]. Similar to the other systems, because these organoids recapitulate the main aspects of retinal development, they represent a valuable tool for studying the cellular mechanisms driving retinal morphogenesis, and perhaps for future treatment of retinal degeneration.

3 Cancer Models

As discussed above, cancer cell lines helped to establish initial 2D culture techniques; however, while valuable resources, they represent only a subclone of the original tumor and have adapted to growth in artificial conditions. To better understand cancer biology and improve preclinical translation into effective therapies, cancer patients are in need of more faithful model systems. Beyond cancer cell lines, patient derived xenografts (PDXs) from primary human tumors have also become a fundamental tool in cancer research and drug discovery [38, 39]. However, additional preclinical cancer models are necessary to overcome the limitations between cell lines, a simple but facile model for high-throughput screening, and PDXs, more complicated and costly, but physiologically relevant.

3D culture of cancer cells as epithelial organoids can generate cellular structures that recapitulate the tissue organization, functional differentiation and the chemical and mechanical signals of the original tumor tissue [20]. Indeed, because cancer organoids can theoretically be derived from tumor tissue for each individual patient, they represent an attractive ex vivo assay to study human cancer biology [40]. Short-term organoid cultures contain most of the components of the original tissue, including tumor cells, endothelial and immune cells and fibroblasts. Thus, they represent an attractive model to recapitulate the human tumor biology, enabling the interactions between neoplastic cells together with extracellular matrix, tumour vasculature and immune cells. Moreover, because cancer cells usually can grow independently of niche factors, the culture conditions of cancer organoids are less stringent when compared with wild-type organoids. For example, the Hans Clevers laboratory successfully generated primary patient-derived organoids from cancerous colon and could maintain them in long-term culture [20].

In addition to their use for the study of human tumor biology, cancer organoids have also a potential role as an ex vivo screening platform for testing efficacy and toxicity of drug compounds. These cultures are established in a relatively short time

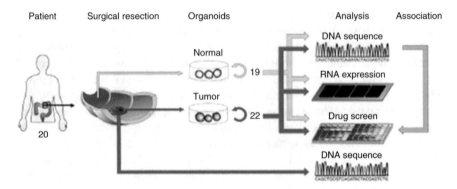

Fig. 2 Overview of the procedure to perform high-throughput screens using organoids derived from primary tissue. Genomic characterization, RNA analysis and high-throughput drug screening of 3D organoids cultures derived from healthy and tumor tissue to identify gene-drug associations that may facilitate personalized therapy

frame, are easy to manipulate and allow high-throughput screens (Fig. 2—reprint with permission). Importantly, human cancer organoids retain the heterogeneity of genetic alterations present in patient samples, reflecting genetic lesions and gene expression patterns. For example, organoid cultures from colorectal cancer have been successfully established from biopsies of metastases with preservation of the genetic diversity. Detailed genetic analysis further demonstrated that these organoids reflect the metastasis from which they were derived [41]. Using a 3D organoid system, Gao et al established long term organoid cultures derived from biopsy specimens and circulating tumor cells from patients with advanced prostate cancer. Of note, these cancer organoid lines recapitulated the molecular diversity of prostate cancer subtypes and represent a powerful genetically manipulatable model for drug testing in vitro and in vivo [40].

Notably, Hans Clevers and colleagues recently reported the establishment of tumor organoid cultures from 20 consecutive patients with colorectal cancer, fact that they called a "living organoid biobank". Interestingly, these organoids closely recapitulated the properties of the original tumors. Gene expression analysis showed that this organoid biobank represented the main colorectal cancer molecular subtypes. Importantly, they successfully developed a high-throughput drug screen in order to identify clinical biomarkers of response using cancer organoids. To this aim, they correlated drug sensitivity with genomic features to identify molecular signatures associated with altered drug response [42]. Similarly, together with the Tuveson laboratory, they established the feasibility of compiling a tissue bank of mouse and human ductal pancreatic cancer organoids, which recapitulated known alterations and enabled proteomic discovery of novel factors that promote pancreatic cancer progression [43].

Interestingly, another recent approach successfully showed that colorectal cancer can be modeled through genetic engineering of human organoids from normal colon tissue. Toshiro Sato and colleagues recently used the CRISPR-Cas9 genome-editing system to introduce multiple mutations into organoids derived from normal human intestinal epithelium. Organoids engineered to express several mutations in tumor suppressor genes common in colorectal cancer grew independently of niche factors in vitro and formed tumors after implantation in mice [44]. Additionally, cancer organoids could be generated following introduction of four of the most commonly mutated colorectal cancer genes (*APC*, *TP53*, *KRAS* and *SMAD4*) in cultured human intestinal stem cells [45]. These mutant organoids grew independently of niche factors and upper xenotransplantation into mice also generated tumors with features of invasive carcinoma. Other groups have been able to induce oncogenic transformation of mouse primary gastric, pancreatic and colon organoids [46]. Pancreatic and gastric organoids showed dysplasia after the expression of $KRAS^{G12D}$, *TP53* loss or both, generating adenocarcinomas after in vivo transplantation. In contrast, primary colon organoids required the mutation of *APC*, *TP53*, *KRAS* and *SMAD4* to induce an invasive adenocarcinoma

In sum, the development of organoid culture technology has enabled the unprecedented opportunity to study primary tumors ex vivo, and to model genetic cancer progression in a more physiologic fashion.

4 Perspectives

It is clear that much remains to be learned about human developmental biology, and the ability to recapitulate organ development outside of the body will have major ramifications of our understanding of normal physiology. In addition, much excitement exists regarding the potential for therapeutic tissue regeneration, although multiple hurdles still remain and will require effective engraftment of organoids back into the host. While cancer organoids also represent an impressive technology to grow tumors ex vivo, important limitations must also still be overcome. In particular, organoid technologies largely focus on the tumor epithelial specific component and not the tumor microenvironment, which is lost over time in culture. However, increasing evidence supports a critical role of the tumor microenvironment in shaping cancer progression and therapeutic response [47–49]. Indeed, tumor formation and progression involves the co-evolution of cancer cells together with the extracellular matrix, endothelial and immune cells and fibroblasts. A continuous interaction exists between tumor cells and non-tumor cell components through direct cell contact or by the secretion of signaling factors such as cytokines, chemokines and growth factors [50, 51]. It is also becoming increasingly clear that the tumor microenvironment can significantly affect the response to anticancer drugs. The recent identification of mechanisms of therapeutic resistance affecting not only the tumor cells, but also their environment, indicates the importance of the study of tumor cell extrinsic compartments on drug resistance [52, 53]. Thus, an important need exists for more sophisticated pre-clinical cancer models that recapitulate human tumor biology and predict response and resistance to cytotoxic or targeted cancer therapies.

As discussed in other chapters, microfluidic culture systems have been developed and are being optimized to recapitulate the tumor microenvironment [54].

This novel microfluidic 3D cell culture technology efficiently incorporates an extracellular matrix (e.g. collagen, matrigel, or fibrin), with co-culture to enable cell-cell interactions that reflect the endothelial and/or immune-cancer cell interface, and allowing controlled analysis of growth factor and cytokine mediated effects. Therefore, this 3D system more closely recapitulates cancer cell behavior in the extracellular matrix, capturing features of the tumor microenvironment and, of note, enabling inhibitor studies in a more physiologic environment. Combining organoid culture with these more complex ex vivo systems rather than traditional well-based matrigel culture would enable more elegant studies of interactions with tumor endothelium and secreted factors that influence behavior in vivo. Hence, 3D microfluidic technologies represent a powerful platform to co-culture patient-derived cancer organoids with stromal, vascular and/or immune cells in order to accurately model tumor complexity and heterogeneity (Fig. 3). Even more importantly, given the emergence of immunotherapy, the ability to culture tumors ex vivo and maintain or reintroduce immune cells could have major implications for the exploding field of immuno-oncology. Since several of these microfluidic technologies enable testing the effects of specific drugs, antibodies, and cytokines [55, 56], these technologies will likely facilitate study of immune directed cancer therapies and a manner not previously possible, and perhaps may ultimately provide a platform for personalizing immunotherapy.

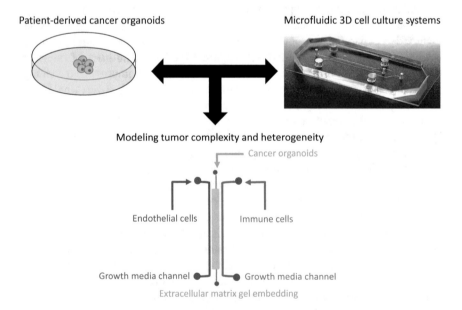

Fig. 3 Modeling tumor complexity and heterogeneity using microfluidic 3D cell culture technology. Microfluidic 3D culture systems represent a powerful platform to co-culture patient-derived organoids with stromal, vascular and/or immune cells in order to recapitulate the tumor microenvironment, enabling more complex studies of interaction with tumor endothelium and secreted factors that influence tumor behavior *in vivo*

References

1. Hayflick L, Moorhead PS (1961) The serial cultivation of human diploid cell strains. Exp Cell Res 25:585–621
2. Bodnar AG, Ouellette M, Frolkis M, Holt SE, Chiu CP, Morin GB, Harley CB, Shay JW, Lichtsteiner S, Wright WE (1998) Extension of life-span by introduction of telomerase into normal human cells. Science 279(5349):349–352
3. Kiyono T, Foster SA, Koop JI, McDougall JK, Galloway DA, Klingelhutz AJ (1998) Both Rb/p16INK4a inactivation and telomerase activity are required to immortalize human epithelial cells. Nature 396(6706):84–88. doi:10.1038/23962
4. Hahn WC, Counter CM, Lundberg AS, Beijersbergen RL, Brooks MW, Weinberg RA (1999) Creation of human tumour cells with defined genetic elements. Nature 400(6743):464–468. doi:10.1038/22780
5. Tahara H, Yasui W, Tahara E, Fujimoto J, Ito K, Tamai K, Nakayama J, Ishikawa F, Tahara E, Ide T (1999) Immuno-histochemical detection of human telomerase catalytic component, hTERT, in human colorectal tumor and non-tumor tissue sections. Oncogene 18(8):1561–1567. doi:10.1038/sj.onc.1202458
6. Schepers AG, Vries R, van den Born M, van de Wetering M, Clevers H (2011) Lgr5 intestinal stem cells have high telomerase activity and randomly segregate their chromosomes. EMBO J 30(6):1104–1109. doi:10.1038/emboj.2011.26
7. Korinek V, Barker N, Moerer P, van Donselaar E, Huls G, Peters PJ, Clevers H (1998) Depletion of epithelial stem-cell compartments in the small intestine of mice lacking Tcf-4. Nat Genet 19(4):379–383. doi:10.1038/1270
8. Barker N, van Es JH, Kuipers J, Kujala P, van den Born M, Cozijnsen M, Haegebarth A, Korving J, Begthel H, Peters PJ, Clevers H (2007) Identification of stem cells in small intestine and colon by marker gene Lgr5. Nature 449(7165):1003–1007. doi:10.1038/nature06196
9. Sato T, Vries RG, Snippert HJ, van de Wetering M, Barker N, Stange DE, van Es JH, Abo A, Kujala P, Peters PJ, Clevers H (2009) Single Lgr5 stem cells build crypt-villus structures in vitro without a mesenchymal niche. Nature 459(7244):262–265. doi:10.1038/nature07935
10. Watanabe K, Kamiya D, Nishiyama A, Katayama T, Nozaki S, Kawasaki H, Watanabe Y, Mizuseki K, Sasai Y (2005) Directed differentiation of telencephalic precursors from embryonic stem cells. Nat Neurosci 8(3):288–296. doi:10.1038/nn1402
11. Eiraku M, Watanabe K, Matsuo-Takasaki M, Kawada M, Yonemura S, Matsumura M, Wataya T, Nishiyama A, Muguruma K, Sasai Y (2008) Self-organized formation of polarized cortical tissues from ESCs and its active manipulation by extrinsic signals. Cell Stem Cell 3(5):519–532. doi:10.1016/j.stem.2008.09.002
12. Eiraku M, Takata N, Ishibashi H, Kawada M, Sakakura E, Okuda S, Sekiguchi K, Adachi T, Sasai Y (2011) Self-organizing optic-cup morphogenesis in three-dimensional culture. Nature 472(7341):51–56. doi:10.1038/nature09941
13. Xinaris C, Benedetti V, Rizzo P, Abbate M, Corna D, Azzollini N, Conti S, Unbekandt M, Davies JA, Morigi M, Benigni A, Remuzzi G (2012) In vivo maturation of functional renal organoids formed from embryonic cell suspensions. J Am Soc Nephrol 23(11):1857–1868. doi:10.1681/ASN.2012050505
14. Zimmermann B (1987) Lung organoid culture. Differentiation 36(1):86–109
15. Levy E, Delvin E, Menard D, Beaulieu JF (2009) Functional development of human fetal gastrointestinal tract. Methods Mol Biol 550:205–224. doi:10.1007/978-1-60327-009-0_13
16. Nakano T, Ando S, Takata N, Kawada M, Muguruma K, Sekiguchi K, Saito K, Yonemura S, Eiraku M, Sasai Y (2012) Self-formation of optic cups and storable stratified neural retina from human ESCs. Cell Stem Cell 10(6):771–785. doi:10.1016/j.stem.2012.05.009

17. Lancaster MA, Renner M, Martin CA, Wenzel D, Bicknell LS, Hurles ME, Homfray T, Penninger JM, Jackson AP, Knoblich JA (2013) Cerebral organoids model human brain development and microcephaly. Nature 501(7467):373–379. doi:10.1038/nature12517

18. Yui S, Nakamura T, Sato T, Nemoto Y, Mizutani T, Zheng X, Ichinose S, Nagaishi T, Okamoto R, Tsuchiya K, Clevers H, Watanabe M (2012) Functional engraftment of colon epithelium expanded in vitro from a single adult Lgr5(+) stem cell. Nat Med 18(4):618–623. doi:10.1038/nm.2695

19. Sato T, van Es JH, Snippert HJ, Stange DE, Vries RG, van den Born M, Barker N, Shroyer NF, van de Wetering M, Clevers H (2011) Paneth cells constitute the niche for Lgr5 stem cells in intestinal crypts. Nature 469(7330):415–418. doi:10.1038/nature09637

20. Sato T, Stange DE, Ferrante M, Vries RG, Van Es JH, Van den Brink S, Van Houdt WJ, Pronk A, Van Gorp J, Siersema PD, Clevers H (2011) Long-term expansion of epithelial organoids from human colon, adenoma, adenocarcinoma, and Barrett's epithelium. Gastroenterology 141(5):1762–1772. doi:10.1053/j.gastro.2011.07.050

21. Spence JR, Mayhew CN, Rankin SA, Kuhar MF, Vallance JE, Tolle K, Hoskins EE, Kalinichenko VV, Wells SI, Zorn AM, Shroyer NF, Wells JM (2011) Directed differentiation of human pluripotent stem cells into intestinal tissue in vitro. Nature 470(7332):105–109. doi:10.1038/nature09691

22. Watson CL, Mahe MM, Munera J, Howell JC, Sundaram N, Poling HM, Schweitzer JI, Vallance JE, Mayhew CN, Sun Y, Grabowski G, Finkbeiner SR, Spence JR, Shroyer NF, Wells JM, Helmrath MA (2014) An in vivo model of human small intestine using pluripotent stem cells. Nat Med 20(11):1310–1314. doi:10.1038/nm.3737

23. McCracken KW, Cata EM, Crawford CM, Sinagoga KL, Schumacher M, Rockich BE, Tsai YH, Mayhew CN, Spence JR, Zavros Y, Wells JM (2014) Modelling human development and disease in pluripotent stem-cell-derived gastric organoids. Nature 516(7531):400–404. doi:10.1038/nature13863

24. Weiss P, Taylor AC (1960) Reconstitution of complete organs from single-cell suspensions of chick embryos in advanced stages of differentiation. Proc Natl Acad Sci U S A 46(9):1177–1185

25. Huch M, Dorrell C, Boj SF, van Es JH, Li VS, van de Wetering M, Sato T, Hamer K, Sasaki N, Finegold MJ, Haft A, Vries RG, Grompe M, Clevers H (2013) In vitro expansion of single Lgr5+ liver stem cells induced by Wnt-driven regeneration. Nature 494(7436):247–250. doi:10.1038/nature11826

26. Huch M, Gehart H, van Boxtel R, Hamer K, Blokzijl F, Verstegen MM, Ellis E, van Wenum M, Fuchs SA, de Ligt J, van de Wetering M, Sasaki N, Boers SJ, Kemperman H, de Jonge J, Ijzermans JN, Nieuwenhuis EE, Hoekstra R, Strom S, Vries RR, van der Laan LJ, Cuppen E, Clevers H (2015) Long-term culture of genome-stable bipotent stem cells from adult human liver. Cell 160(1–2):299–312. doi:10.1016/j.cell.2014.11.050

27. Takebe T, Sekine K, Enomura M, Koike H, Kimura M, Ogaeri T, Zhang RR, Ueno Y, Zheng YW, Koike N, Aoyama S, Adachi Y, Taniguchi H (2013) Vascularized and functional human liver from an iPSC-derived organ bud transplant. Nature 499(7459):481–484. doi:10.1038/nature12271

28. Auerbach R, Grobstein C (1958) Inductive interaction of embryonic tissues after dissociation and reaggregation. Exp Cell Res 15(2):384–397

29. Xia Y, Nivet E, Sancho-Martinez I, Gallegos T, Suzuki K, Okamura D, Wu MZ, Dubova I, Esteban CR, Montserrat N, Campistol JM, Izpisua Belmonte JC (2013) Directed differentiation of human pluripotent cells to ureteric bud kidney progenitor-like cells. Nat Cell Biol 15(12):1507–1515. doi:10.1038/ncb2872

30. Taguchi A, Kaku Y, Ohmori T, Sharmin S, Ogawa M, Sasaki H, Nishinakamura R (2014) Redefining the in vivo origin of metanephric nephron progenitors enables generation of complex kidney structures from pluripotent stem cells. Cell Stem Cell 14(1):53–67. doi:10.1016/j.stem.2013.11.010

31. Takasato M, Er PX, Becroft M, Vanslambrouck JM, Stanley EG, Elefanty AG, Little MH (2014) Directing human embryonic stem cell differentiation towards a renal lineage generates a self-organizing kidney. Nat Cell Biol 16(1):118–126. doi:10.1038/ncb2894

32. Ishii K (1966) Reconstruction of dissociated chick brain cells in rotation-mediated culture. Cytologia (Tokyo) 31(1):89–98
33. Conti L, Cattaneo E (2010) Neural stem cell systems: physiological players or in vitro entities? Nat Rev Neurosci 11(3):176–187. doi:10.1038/nrn2761
34. Kadoshima T, Sakaguchi H, Nakano T, Soen M, Ando S, Eiraku M, Sasai Y (2013) Self-organization of axial polarity, inside-out layer pattern, and species-specific progenitor dynamics in human ES cell-derived neocortex. Proc Natl Acad Sci U S A 110(50):20284–20289. doi:10.1073/pnas.1315710110
35. Danjo T, Eiraku M, Muguruma K, Watanabe K, Kawada M, Yanagawa Y, Rubenstein JL, Sasai Y (2011) Subregional specification of embryonic stem cell-derived ventral telencephalic tissues by timed and combinatory treatment with extrinsic signals. J Neurosci 31(5):1919–1933. doi:10.1523/JNEUROSCI.5128-10.2011
36. Su HL, Muguruma K, Matsuo-Takasaki M, Kengaku M, Watanabe K, Sasai Y (2006) Generation of cerebellar neuron precursors from embryonic stem cells. Dev Biol 290(2):287–296. doi:10.1016/j.ydbio.2005.11.010
37. Layer PG, Robitzki A, Rothermel A, Willbold E (2002) Of layers and spheres: the reaggregate approach in tissue engineering. Trends Neurosci 25(3):131–134
38. Bertotti A, Migliardi G, Galimi F, Sassi F, Torti D, Isella C, Cora D, Di Nicolantonio F, Buscarino M, Petti C, Ribero D, Russolillo N, Muratore A, Massucco P, Pisacane A, Molinaro L, Valtorta E, Sartore-Bianchi A, Risio M, Capussotti L, Gambacorta M, Siena S, Medico E, Sapino A, Marsoni S, Comoglio PM, Bardelli A, Trusolino L (2011) A molecularly annotated platform of patient-derived xenografts ("xenopatients") identifies HER2 as an effective therapeutic target in cetuximab-resistant colorectal cancer. Cancer Discov 1(6):508–523. doi:10.1158/2159-8290.CD-11-0109
39. Gao H, Korn JM, Ferretti S, Monahan JE, Wang Y, Singh M, Zhang C, Schnell C, Yang G, Zhang Y, Balbin OA, Barbe S, Cai H, Casey F, Chatterjee S, Chiang DY, Chuai S, Cogan SM, Collins SD, Dammassa E, Ebel N, Embry M, Green J, Kauffmann A, Kowal C, Leary RJ, Lehar J, Liang Y, Loo A, Lorenzana E, Robert McDonald E 3rd, McLaughlin ME, Merkin J, Meyer R, Naylor TL, Patawaran M, Reddy A, Roelli C, Ruddy DA, Salangsang F, Santacroce F, Singh AP, Tang Y, Tinetto W, Tobler S, Velazquez R, Venkatesan K, Von Arx F, Wang HQ, Wang Z, Wiesmann M, Wyss D, Xu F, Bitter H, Atadja P, Lees E, Hofmann F, Li E, Keen N, Cozens R, Jensen MR, Pryer NK, Williams JA, Sellers WR (2015) High-throughput screening using patient-derived tumor xenografts to predict clinical trial drug response. Nat Med 21(11):1318–1325. doi:10.1038/nm.3954
40. Gao D, Vela I, Sboner A, Iaquinta PJ, Karthaus WR, Gopalan A, Dowling C, Wanjala JN, Undvall EA, Arora VK, Wongvipat J, Kossai M, Ramazanoglu S, Barboza LP, Di W, Cao Z, Zhang QF, Sirota I, Ran L, MacDonald TY, Beltran H, Mosquera JM, Touijer KA, Scardino PT, Laudone VP, Curtis KR, Rathkopf DE, Morris MJ, Danila DC, Slovin SF, Solomon SB, Eastham JA, Chi P, Carver B, Rubin MA, Scher HI, Clevers H, Sawyers CL, Chen Y (2014) Organoid cultures derived from patients with advanced prostate cancer. Cell 159(1):176–187. doi:10.1016/j.cell.2014.08.016
41. Weeber F, van de Wetering M, Hoogstraat M, Dijkstra KK, Krijgsman O, Kuilman T, Gadellaa-van Hooijdonk CG, van der Velden DL, Peeper DS, Cuppen EP, Vries RG, Clevers H, Voest EE (2015) Preserved genetic diversity in organoids cultured from biopsies of human colorectal cancer metastases. Proc Natl Acad Sci U S A 112(43):13308–13311. doi:10.1073/pnas.1516689112
42. van de Wetering M, Francies HE, Francis JM, Bounova G, Iorio F, Pronk A, van Houdt W, van Gorp J, Taylor-Weiner A, Kester L, McLaren-Douglas A, Blokker J, Jaksani S, Bartfeld S, Volckman R, van Sluis P, Li VS, Seepo S, Sekhar Pedamallu C, Cibulskis K, Carter SL, McKenna A, Lawrence MS, Lichtenstein L, Stewart C, Koster J, Versteeg R, van Oudenaarden A, Saez-Rodriguez J, Vries RG, Getz G, Wessels L, Stratton MR, McDermott U, Meyerson M, Garnett MJ, Clevers H (2015) Prospective derivation of a living organoid biobank of colorectal cancer patients. Cell 161(4):933–945. doi:10.1016/j.cell.2015.03.053
43. Boj SF, Hwang CI, Baker LA, Chio II, Engle DD, Corbo V, Jager M, Ponz-Sarvise M, Tiriac H, Spector MS, Gracanin A, Oni T, Yu KH, van Boxtel R, Huch M, Rivera KD, Wilson JP,

Feigin ME, Ohlund D, Handly-Santana A, Ardito-Abraham CM, Ludwig M, Elyada E, Alagesan B, Biffi G, Yordanov GN, Delcuze B, Creighton B, Wright K, Park Y, Morsink FH, Molenaar IQ, Borel Rinkes IH, Cuppen E, Hao Y, Jin Y, Nijman IJ, Iacobuzio-Donahue C, Leach SD, Pappin DJ, Hammell M, Klimstra DS, Basturk O, Hruban RH, Offerhaus GJ, Vries RG, Clevers H, Tuveson DA (2015) Organoid models of human and mouse ductal pancreatic cancer. Cell 160(1–2):324–338. doi:10.1016/j.cell.2014.12.021

44. Matano M, Date S, Shimokawa M, Takano A, Fujii M, Ohta Y, Watanabe T, Kanai T, Sato T (2015) Modeling colorectal cancer using CRISPR-Cas9-mediated engineering of human intestinal organoids. Nat Med 21(3):256–262. doi:10.1038/nm.3802
45. Drost J, van Jaarsveld RH, Ponsioen B, Zimberlin C, van Boxtel R, Buijs A, Sachs N, Overmeer RM, Offerhaus GJ, Begthel H, Korving J, van de Wetering M, Schwank G, Logtenberg M, Cuppen E, Snippert HJ, Medema JP, Kops GJ, Clevers H (2015) Sequential cancer mutations in cultured human intestinal stem cells. Nature 521(7550):43–47. doi:10.1038/nature14415
46. Li X, Nadauld L, Ootani A, Corney DC, Pai RK, Gevaert O, Cantrell MA, Rack PG, Neal JT, Chan CW, Yeung T, Gong X, Yuan J, Wilhelmy J, Robine S, Attardi LD, Plevritis SK, Hung KE, Chen CZ, Ji HP, Kuo CJ (2014) Oncogenic transformation of diverse gastrointestinal tissues in primary organoid culture. Nat Med 20(7):769–777. doi:10.1038/nm.3585
47. Lu H, Clauser KR, Tam WL, Frose J, Ye X, Eaton EN, Reinhardt F, Donnenberg VS, Bhargava R, Carr SA, Weinberg RA (2014) A breast cancer stem cell niche supported by juxtacrine signalling from monocytes and macrophages. Nat Cell Biol 16(11):1105–1117. doi:10.1038/ncb3041
48. Orimo A, Gupta PB, Sgroi DC, Arenzana-Seisdedos F, Delaunay T, Naeem R, Carey VJ, Richardson AL, Weinberg RA (2005) Stromal fibroblasts present in invasive human breast carcinomas promote tumor growth and angiogenesis through elevated SDF-1/CXCL12 secretion. Cell 121(3):335–348. doi:10.1016/j.cell.2005.02.034
49. Karnoub AE, Dash AB, Vo AP, Sullivan A, Brooks MW, Bell GW, Richardson AL, Polyak K, Tubo R, Weinberg RA (2007) Mesenchymal stem cells within tumour stroma promote breast cancer metastasis. Nature 449(7162):557–563. doi:10.1038/nature06188
50. Malanchi I, Santamaria-Martinez A, Susanto E, Peng H, Lehr HA, Delaloye JF, Huelsken J (2012) Interactions between cancer stem cells and their niche govern metastatic colonization. Nature 481(7379):85–89. doi:10.1038/nature10694
51. Hanahan D, Coussens LM (2012) Accessories to the crime: functions of cells recruited to the tumor microenvironment. Cancer Cell 21(3):309–322. doi:10.1016/j.ccr.2012.02.022
52. Meads MB, Gatenby RA, Dalton WS (2009) Environment-mediated drug resistance: a major contributor to minimal residual disease. Nat Rev Cancer 9(9):665–674. doi:10.1038/nrc2714
53. Nakasone ES, Askautrud HA, Kees T, Park JH, Plaks V, Ewald AJ, Fein M, Rasch MG, Tan YX, Qiu J, Park J, Sinha P, Bissell MJ, Frengen E, Werb Z, Egeblad M (2012) Imaging tumor-stroma interactions during chemotherapy reveals contributions of the microenvironment to resistance. Cancer Cell 21(4):488–503. doi:10.1016/j.ccr.2012.02.017
54. Aref AR, Huang RY, Yu W, Chua KN, Sun W, Tu TY, Bai J, Sim WJ, Zervantonakis IK, Thiery JP, Kamm RD (2013) Screening therapeutic EMT blocking agents in a three-dimensional microenvironment. Integr Biol (Camb) 5(2):381–389. doi:10.1039/c2ib20209c
55. Zhu Z, Aref AR, Cohoon TJ, Barbie TU, Imamura Y, Yang S, Moody SE, Shen RR, Schinzel AC, Thai TC, Reibel JB, Tamayo P, Godfrey JT, Qian ZR, Page AN, Maciag K, Chan EM, Silkworth W, Labowsky MT, Rozhansky L, Mesirov JP, Gillanders WE, Ogino S, Hacohen N, Gaudet S, Eck MJ, Engelman JA, Corcoran RB, Wong KK, Hahn WC, Barbie DA (2014) Inhibition of KRAS-driven tumorigenicity by interruption of an autocrine cytokine circuit. Cancer Discov 4(4):452–465. doi:10.1158/2159-8290.CD-13-0646
56. Barbie TU, Alexe G, Aref AR, Li S, Zhu Z, Zhang X, Imamura Y, Thai TC, Huang Y, Bowden M, Herndon J, Cohoon TJ, Fleming T, Tamayo P, Mesirov JP, Ogino S, Wong KK, Ellis MJ, Hahn WC, Barbie DA, Gillanders WE (2014) Targeting an IKBKE cytokine network impairs triple-negative breast cancer growth. J Clin Invest 124(12):5411–5423. doi:10.1172/JCI75661

Microfluidics and Future of Cancer Diagnostics

Samira Jamalian, Mohammad Jafarnejad, and Amir R. Aref

1 Components of the Tumor Microenvironment

Initiation, progression, and metastasis of solid tumors are strikingly affected by interactions of tumor cells with their surrounding stroma. Additionally, these interactions play a major role in development of drug resistance in solid tumors. Interactions of tumor stroma and leukocytes influence anti-tumor immunity and response to immunotherapies. Thus, there is growing interest in understanding the tumor-stromal interactions within the tumor microenvironment (TME) and how they contribute to tumor progression [1].

Cancer cell division and metastasis results in alteration in the TME at the molecular, cellular, and physical level. The resulting tumor microenvironment thus contains a variety of non-malignant cells (e.g., blood endothelial cells, lymphatic endothelial cells, mesenchymal cells, and immune cells) as well as extra cellular matrix and inflammatory mediators secreted by the present cells [2–4]. It is known that solid tumors have incomplete basal lamina, resulting in close interactions between the TME and tumor cells. Dynamic interaction with TME begins at early stages of cancer cell malignant growth and continues as the disease progresses. Thus TME affects cancer cell growth and metastasis as well as therapeutic outcome [5–7].

TME composition varies across different cancer types, but there are similar components across almost all solid tumors. Most tumors have disorganized and leaky vasculature, they are infiltrated by innate and adaptive immune cells that could have

S. Jamalian (✉) • M. Jafarnejad
Department of Bioengineering, Imperial College London,
South Kensington Campus, London SW7 2AZ, UK
e-mail: samira.jamalian12@imperial.ac.uk

A.R. Aref (✉)
Department of Medical Oncology, Dana-Farber Cancer Institute, Boston, MA 02215, USA
e-mail: amirr_aref@dfci.harvard.edu

© Springer International Publishing Switzerland 2017
A.R. Aref, D. Barbie (eds.), *Ex Vivo Engineering of the Tumor Microenvironment*,
Cancer Drug Discovery and Development, DOI 10.1007/978-3-319-45397-2_4

protumor and antitumor functionality. Apart from immune cells, TME also contains a variety of non-hematopoietic cells such as blood endothelial cells, lymphatic endothelial cells, mesenchymal stem cells or their differentiated forms, cancer associated fibroblasts, and pericytes. Other less abundant cell types include neurons, fibrocytes, adipocytes, and follicular dendritic cells [1].

1.1 Immune Microenvironment

The immune system can recognize tumor cells and remove them from the body either naturally or via therapeutic intervention. To achieve anti-tumor immunity certain events in the cancer-immunity cycle need to occur [8]. The cycle begins when tumor cells released by antigens are picked up by dendritic cells (DCs) and transported to lymph nodes (LN) via lymph vessels. When they arrive to the tumor draining LNs, DCs activate antigen specific CD4+ and CD8+ T cells by presenting tumor derived peptides on MHC molecules. When activated, T cells enter the blood stream from LN and circulate in the body. In the next step, T cells extravasate through the blood stream into the tumor environment. Chemokine gradients and adhesion molecules are important for this step. T cells can detect cells that present their cognate antigen in the TME and destroy them. Additional antigens are released following cancer cell death. A new cancer-immunity cycle begins when these antigens themselves are transported to the LN.

The ideal condition would be that cytotoxic immune cells remove all cancerous cells and prevent future tumor progress by building tumor specific immunological memory. But T cell immunity can be impaired at any of the steps described above, due to the complex TME-immune system interactions. Altered or overexpressed genes make up the antigens released by the tumors, this results in self-antigen presentation in the LN, which in turn causes peripheral tolerance. Factors such as chemokine gradients or disorganized vascular networks can be an obstacle for activated T cells to reach the tumor bed. Such self-antigen presentation in the LN can result in peripheral tolerance. Within the tumor itself, inhibitor cells and molecules can disrupt T cell functionality [9].

Immune checkpoint inhibitors have shown great promise in treating a variety of cancers. These immunotherapies remove the break of the immune system by blocking molecules such as cytotoxic T lymphocyte antigen 4 (CTLA4), programmed cell death protein 1 (PD1), and programmed cell death ligand 1 (PDL1). For example, PDL1 when bound to PD1 on activated T cells, inhibits T cell activation and survival, suppressing immune response to tumors. Antibodies that block PD1-PDL1 increase tumor cell killing via CD8+ T cell. Despite the great promise of immune checkpoint inhibitors, not all patients within a given diagnostic group respond to such immunotherapies. It is crucial to identify immunosuppressive mechanisms within the TME that can prevent responsiveness to therapy to increase the patient population that can benefit from immunotherapeutics [1, 10–12].

1.2   Flow in TME and the Effects on the Tumor Stroma

Recent studies of antibodies that block the inhibitory molecules CTLA4, PD1, PDL1 have demonstrated that lymph vessels within the TME play a major role in tumor metastasis. Fluid balance between interstitium and lymph is disrupted in solid tumors [13–15]. The rapid growth of tumor mass and resultant hypoxia together promote angiogenesis [16]. Tumor angiogenesis creates leaky tumor vessels and causes macromolecules (e.g., albumin) build up in tumor tissue. Simultaneously, remodeling of ECM at the tumor margin generates mechanical stress [17, 18]. Together with leaky vessels, this results in increased interstitial fluid pressure (IFP). Tumor IFP can rise to the level of capillary pressure (10–40 mmHg) [14, 16, 18, 19], whereas tissue pressures are usually very low or even negative (−2–0 mmHg) [20]. Anti-angiogenic agents have been shown to decrease tumor IFP [19, 21]. Increased IFP creates pressure gradients at the tumor margin [22, 23] that produces higher interstitial flow in the tumor stroma and surrounding lymph vessels. In addition to promoting angiogenesis, tumors also induce lymphangiogenesis. Invasion, metastasis, and poor prognosis are associated with increased lymphangiogenesis and higher expression of VEGFC and VEGFD. Raju et al. found that increased IFP resulted in higher lymphatic density, and in turn cancer progression in rats with squamous cell carcinoma [24]. Additionally, high interstitial flow exerts mechanical stress on the ECM and stromal cells [25]. This results in higher expression of TGFβ and its activation as well as differentiation of myofibroblasts resulting in stromal stiffening. Better understanding of the relationship between lymph flow, stromal alterations, and how they contribute to tumor immunity is a step toward development of new immunotherapies [15].

2   Strategies for Studying the Tumor Microenvironment

2.1   Conventional TME Models

Traditional methods for studying cells of TME involve cell culture and use of animal models. Culture methods began primarily by culturing cells on 2D surfaces. It has now become evident that 2D cultures oversimplify the tumor microenvironment and lack physiologic relevance [26]. For example, it has been shown that only cells in 3D culture are round shaped and demonstrate similar clustering as tumors in vivo [27, 28]. Moreover, expression profile of genes involved in important metastatic steps (angiogenesis, cell migration, and invasion) varies in 2D versus 3D cultures. Thus 3D microenvironment of tumors must be included to increase the physiologic relevance of in vitro models [29–33]. 3D cultures could be scaffold free as in tumor spheroids, or scaffold-based [34]. Tumor spheroids have been particularly advantageous for testing chemotherapeutics due to their tumor like features, but have not been widely used in drug discovery yet, mostly due to technical difficulties.

Scaffold-based 3D cultures are useful for studying tumor migration and invasion in the TME [35, 36]. Scaffold material itself can be functionalized to obtain desired chemical and biological characteristics [37]. Scaffold materials and their application in cancer research have been extensively reviewed in the literature [29].

Other popular strategies for studying TME are ex vivo or in vivo models, such as patient derived xenograft (PDX) models. Ex vivo models improve upon 2D cultures by conserving the cell matrix. In these methods, tumor tissue from human or animals is cultured on a porous substrate and embedded in an ECM like matrix [38, 39]. 3D cultures more accurately mimic cell behavior. The disadvantage of ex vivo culture methods is the absence of mechanical forces such as shear stress [29].

Animal models have allowed researchers to predict drug behavior and efficiency and provide the complex tumor environment. However, because the cells are inherently different in animals compared to humans, all cellular functions (metabolism, proliferation, and metastasis) will be inevitably different. The difference in immune function adds to this complexity and reduces the predictive power as well. Moreover, there is growing emphasis on less use of animals as research subject [40, 41].

PDX models improve upon the disadvantage in inherent cell difference by engrafting primary tumor samples onto immune deficient mice, allowing identification of biomarkers of response or resistance to drug. They provide an important tool toward personalization of medicine [42]. PDX models offer significant advances over traditional cancer cell line-based studies, but this model system requires expensive cohorts of immunocompromised mice as well as a long period time to establish sufficient number of tumors. Because of this problem of scale PDX models have limited ability to test multiple drug concentrations and/or combinations. Thus, development of better experimental platforms is required to evaluate response to therapies in real time and further progress toward personalized cancer medicine [42].

2.2 Microfluidic Devices

A critical need exists for physiologically relevant experimental platforms that recapitulate the tumor microenvironment. Some of the main challenges facing conventional culture methods were issues of vascularization in the TME, metabolism and application of mechanical forces. Microfluidic platforms have emerged as powerful tools that allow high levels of control over substrate structure, application of mechanical forces, chemical gradients and can more accurately represent the in vivo TME.

Microfluidic devices provide distinct advantage by enabling interaction between multiple cell types in 3D, they allow real time monitoring of the response to stimulants of interest (e.g., drugs, mechanical forces) and permit control over those stimulants. Thus, microfluidic technologies via their distinct advantages have clear potential for studying the metastatic cascade. Their unique imaging capabilities are specially useful for such studies as well [43, 44]. Metastasis occurs in multiple steps, and is often difficult to observe and track in vivo. Epithelial to mesenchymal transition (EMT), invasion, intravasation, transport of circulating tumor cells

(CTCs), extravasation in other tissues, and eventually forming new masses at the new site are the steps for the metastatic cycle [45]. Special equipment and expertise are required for intravital imaging in vivo and the depth in which the organ is located might negatively affect image resolution. Another issue is the scale (number of cells) involved in each metastatic step [46]. If the events of interest are rare occurrences, this poses yet another challenge for in vivo imaging. A critical need exists for thorough understanding of the metastatic cascade, as each step could be targeted for therapeutics to slow down or eliminate metastasis. Microfluidic technologies are increasingly being used to model each of these steps individually.

Intravasation occurs when cancer cells migrate across the endothelium into the blood stream. Extravasation on the other hand is migration from blood circulation to the adjacent tissues. Interaction with blood or endothelial cells is inevitable for some of these steps such as intravasation or extravasation. It is thus evident that presence of endothelium is essential for studying cancer and should be included in microfluidic devices. With this in mind, several investigators have cultured endothelial cells in PDMS microchannels [47–51]. Having the endothelial monolayer while culturing cancer cells in the hydrogel, allowed researchers to study intravasation [48, 50]. For extravasation [47, 49, 51] or adhesion studies [51–53], cancer cells are directly embedded in the channel. Microvascular networks can be formed via self-organization of ECs that are suspended in hydrogel in presence of fibroblasts [54, 55] or mesenchymal stem cells [56]. There is growing interest in using microvascular networks [49, 57–59] as they provide more realistic dimensions, morphology, and permeability relative to in vivo vascular beds [57]. Microvascular networks can be made in well plates, but in the microfluidic devices microvascular networks can be grown in hydrogel supported by the microchannels themselves, this allows the lumen of the vessel to remain open, allowing perfusion through the network. For the purpose of extravasation studies, cancer cells could be introduced to the system as well [57]. In traditional 2D extravasation models (e.g., Boydon chamber) ECs are seeded into a permeable membrane and placed in a well plate, but the problem with this system is imaging. Trasnwells do not allow for high-resolution single cell imaging because of the long distance between the membrane and the objective, microfluidic devices provide a better imaging capability. Additional advantages come from more realistic 3D vessel architecture and EC barrier function [57]. Microfluidic technologies can take advantage of the capabilities of microvascular networks to study EC-cancer cell interaction and dynamics as well as other cell types. As mentioned before, these assays can be used for study of every step of the metastatic cascade.

2.2.1 Cell Migration

Microfluidic devices enable observation of cancer cell dispersion and migration from spheroids to the collagen gel to provide understanding of EMT and invasion [60, 61]. It has been observed that migratory cells express EpCAM on a lower level compared to the cells that remain in the spheroid, suggesting that these cells have undergone EMT, as occurs in vivo. Other studies have shown that an invasive phenotype in breast cancer cells results in collagen remodeling and is promoted by human mammary fibroblasts [62, 63]. Another study observed increased invasion of a cancer cell line into the hydrogel as metastatic potential increased [52]. A similar increase was detected under hypoxia [64] or in presence of CXCL12 or matrix metalloproteinase (MMP) inhibitors.

2.2.2   Intravasation Models

Microfluidic intravasation assays have shown increased cancer cell transmigration across an EC monolayer in the presence of TNF-alpha [48, 50] and macrophages [50], in agreement with in vivo observations [44]. Using a Boyden chamber with microfluidic channels it was shown that luminal and transmural flow increased intravasation through a lymphatic monolayer [65]. Enhanced intravasation was observed under hypoxia in a vascularized spheroid of cancer cells in a well plate [58]. It was reported that the observation depended on transcription factor SLUG, in agreement with in vivo results [66]. It is necessary to repeat these experiments in the advanced microfluidic devices and take advantage of their novel capabilities (e.g., microvascular networks).

2.2.3   Adhesion Models

Adhesion of single cancer cells or cell aggregates onto an EC monolayer in microfluidic devices demonstrated that E-selectin expression in HUVEC, CXCL12 [53], and shear stress [49] could mediate adhesion.

2.2.4   Extravasation Models

Observation of extravasation in microfluidic devices has shown that breast cancer cells extravasate within 24 h through the transient gaps between the ECs of a microvascular network [47, 57]. Extravasation of tumor cell aggregates on the other hand was followed by irreversible disruption of EC monolayer [51]. Presence of osteo-like cells resulted in increased extravasation rate [67], indicating the preference of breast cancer cells to metastasize in bone (organ selectivity) as has been observed in vivo. An increase in extravasation was also observed by presence of CXCL12 [49]. AMD3100 (which is a CXCR4 receptor antagonist that is currently in clinical trials) blocked extravasation [51]. An alternative method used for studying extravasation is measuring cell deformability through narrow gaps either in 2D or channels filled with hydrogels [68].

Better understanding of micrometastasis events following extravasation is of high importance. This stage is known to be the least efficient step in metastasis cascade and has a great potential for therapeutic targeting for impeding metastasis. Microvascular networks in well plates have been used to study processes beyond extravasation [59], and microfluidic platforms have great potential for such studies. Quantification of cancer cell proliferation or invasion in the ECM occurring shortly following extravasation showed that CXCL12 increased the invasion [51]. Currently, only a single study has attempted to investigate multiple metastatic steps in the same microfluidic device. The study combines invasion of cancer cells from hydrogel and then adhesion to a monolayer of ECs [52].

Addressing organ selectivity in metastasis is another important challenge [69]. Understanding the organ-specific cancer cell interactions can help develop new therapeutics for preventing metastasis in secondary organs. As cancer cells interact with their environment, they interact with organ-specific cells, resulting in organ selectivity [5, 70, 71]. Microfluidic devices are well suited for studying these interactions because they allow control over distribution of cells of different types to resemble organ specific cells in vivo. Organ specific phenomen a have been studied using organ specific cell types [67] or chemokines [51] in microfluidic devices. Another study modeled the air-liquid interface to represent the pulmonary airways [72]. Microfluidic assays have the potential to grow in terms of complexity by including other stromal cells or immune cells to study their role in metastasis as well as response to therapeutics.

2.2.5 Epithelial-Mesenchymal Transition Model

A majority of cancers are of epithelial origin, and the progression of carcinoma has been hypothesized to involve epithelial–mesenchymal transition (EMT). EMT has also been implicated in the formation of tumor-initiating or cancer stem cells and in drug resistance. Aref et al. demonstrated a tumor microenvironment model based on a microfluidic device (Fig. 1) capable of (1) recapitulating the physical and

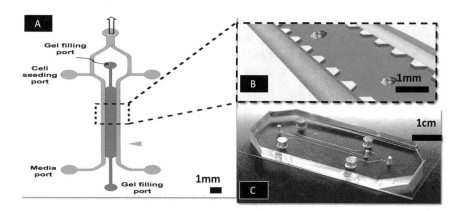

Fig. 1 Schematic and photograph of a 3D co-culture microfluidic device. (**a**) Schematic diagram of the layout of the device depicts the inlets for injecting cells, filling with collagen, and replenishing medium. (**b**) Enlarged view of the gel region and the HUVEC-lined channel. Cytokines in conditioned medium from the HUVEC monolayer diffuse into the gel region, triggering spheroids to undergo EMT. (**c**) Photograph of the PDMS-molded device bonded on a glass cover-slip

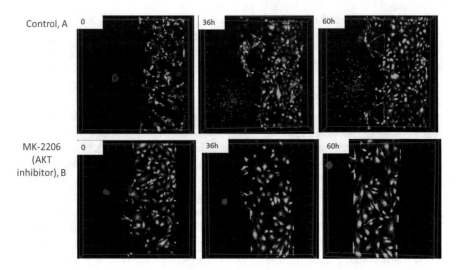

Fig. 2 Fluorescent images in time-series showing A549 cell dissemination in the 3D collagen gel. (**a**) Control condition in the presence of a HUVEC monolayer in the side channel, i.e. 3D co-culture. (**b**) AKT-targeted drug (300 nM of MK-2206) applied in the presence of a HUVEC monolayer. *Red*: nuclei of A549 cells (Human lung cancer cell line); *green*: HUVEC (Color figure online) [73]

biochemical contexts that allows for the manifestation of EMT of cancer cells in 3D, in the presence of human endothelial cells; and (2) quantitatively monitoring the EMT inhibitory effects of drugs [73].

As a step toward a more realistic in vitro assay, they developed a 3D microfluidic system, and accompanying image analysis process to characterize the statistics of anti-metastatic drug responses. Their results confirmed the importance of growing cells in 2D vs. 3D. Furthermore, they demonstrated that presence of other cell types, in this case endothelial cells, can significantly alter the levels of drug required to inhibit EMT (Fig. 2). The system was also used to obtain a mechanistic understanding of cell signaling in early metastasis. These studies therefore offer a new approach in drug screening with the potential to better replicate the in vivo microenvironment.

2.2.6 Cytokines Secretion Model

Models for disease processes are critically important for improving understanding and developing new therapeutics. Microfluidic assays provide unique capabilities for mimicking the local microenvironment in terms of multiple cell types, and for controlling and monitoring chemical gradients and cellular interactions. Zhu and Aref showed that a 3D system more closely recapitulates cancer cell behavior in the extracellular matrix, captures key features of the tumor microenvironment, and also enables inhibitor studies [74]. Incubation of A549 cells with CCL5- and

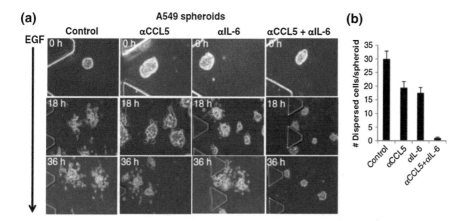

Fig. 3 (**a**) Phase-contrast images of A549 spheroids at 0 (×20), 18, and 36 h (×10) following EGF stimulation (20 ng/mL) ± neutralizing antibodies against CCL5 (100 ng/mL), IL-6 (100 ng/mL), or the combination. (**b**) Mean ± SD number of dispersed cells per spheroid from triplicate devices shown

IL-6–neutralizing antibodies in 2D culture had a minor effect on proliferation (Fig. 3a). In contrast, combined CCL5 and IL-6 blockade completely suppressed A549 cell proliferation in response to EGF in 3D culture, compared with neutralization of either of the cytokines alone (Fig. 3b).

2.2.7 Targeting Cytokines Network in Breast Cancer

The microfluidic technology holds great promise in a variety of settings. A recent study at Dana-Farber Cancer Institute showed that addition of CCL5 and IL-6 to the media in 3D culture models, not only promoted tumor spheroid dispersal but also stimulated proliferation and migration of endothelial cells [75]. These cytokines have been reported in a lung cancer model before.

They reported that in 3D culture, CCL5 and IL-6 not only promoted MDA-MB-468 cell migration and proliferation as effectively as EGF but they also completely rescued the inhibition of spheroid dispersal by CYT387. Taken together, these observations demonstrate that IKBKE-driven CCL5 and IL-6 directly contribute to TNBC migration and proliferation of tumor spheroids, which is disrupted by CYT387 treatment. TBK1/IKBKE-regulated cytokines also influence the tumor microenvironment and angiogenesis in particular. They therefore used another 3D device optimized to study the effects of IKBKE-induced CCL5/IL-6 on HUVEC behavior in collagen (Fig. 4) [76].

2.2.8 Overcome Resistance for the FGFR Inhibitors

Another study conducted by Gray's group combines drug screening and microfluidic technologies to describe a novel kinase inhibitor design strategy that uses a single electrophile to target covalently cysteines located in different positions within

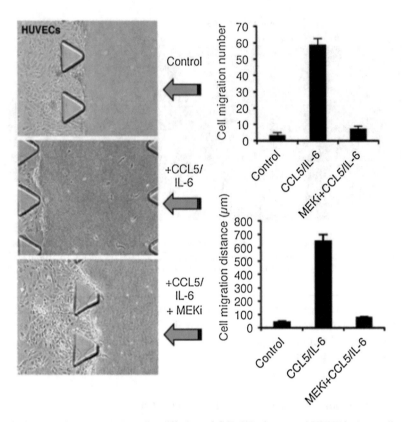

Fig. 4 Compared with control media, diffusion of CCL5/IL-6-attracted HUVECs into collagen (original magnification, ×20) over the course of 24 h. Cotreatment with the MEK inhibitor (MEKi), GSK1120212, at 10 nM strongly inhibited this effect. Mean and SD of cell migration per number from three independent devices are reported

the ATP-binding pocket. Two new generation FGFR inhibitors FIIN-2 and FIIN-3 were evaluated using 3D dispersion assays in a microfluidic device. Compared with conventional 2D assay, the 3D assay creates a 3D microenvironment that allows better evaluation of drugs that inhibit cell migration or epithelial–mesenchymal transition [77].

3 Applications and Opportunities

Immunotherapy has demonstrated striking durable responses in treatment of diverse cancer types. Increasing the number of patients who respond to immunotherapies and improving the therapeutic efficacy using combinatorial therapies are now an important area of focus for this type of therapeutics. It is also crucial to understand the reasons behind responsiveness and unresponsiveness of certain types of cancer to immunotherapy. Deeper understanding of the underlying processes in these areas can accelerate translation of immunotherapies to clinic. A major technological need exists for development of robust models that enable culture of primary human cancers and mimic the principal components of the tumor microenvironment (including the immune environment) [78]. Microfluidic technologies enable characterization of the tumor at the time of diagnosis as well as assessment of its immune environment. This can help identify the type of defense mechanism recruited by the tumor and allow more accurate prediction of tumor response to immunotherapies. The knowledge obtained by such assessments can be used to develop personalized treatment strategies for patients. Microfluidic assays also present a powerful predictive tool for treatment outcome. Implementing patient-derived tumors in vitro more accurately recapitulates major players in the TME, thus the predictions obtained will be more reliable. Furthermore, with microfluidic technology multiple potential therapies and combination therapies can be tested in a rapid and high throughput fashion. This is a powerful tool for guiding treatment and deciding the best possible treatment option for each patient.

Among cancer immunotherapies, immune checkpoint inhibition has been the most successful approach to date [79, 80]. Monoclonal antibodies blocking programmed cell death 1 (PD-1) [81] or its ligand PD-L1 [11] have provided durable treatment for some patients suffering from metastatic melanomas, with higher response rate and fewer side effects compared to cytotoxic T-lymphocyte-associated protein 4 (CTLA-4) blockade [82]. Following the success in metastatic melanoma, immune checkpoint inhibitors have been examined for treatment of several tumor types such as non-small cell lung cancer (NSCLC) and have shown promising results in clinical trials and even received FDA approval in the case of advanced squamous NSCLC (Nivolumab). However, not all patients within a given diagnostic group benefit from treatment with immune checkpoint blockades. Additionally, autoimmune reaction is the main side effect to immune checkpoint inhibitors. Better engineering approaches need to be developed to overcome this challenge. Moreover, we need to be able to recapitulate the tumor immune environment in vitro using patient derived cells. Such microfluidic assays can be recruited to test the efficacy of immune checkpoint blockade therapies alone, or in combination with drugs aimed at immune suppressive pathways in the tumor stroma. Currently, several studies using patient derived cells exist but none include the immune environment [76]. Apart from genetics of the tumor, efficacy of immunotherapy is affected by the components of the tumor microenvironment. The eventual aim is to translate these promising approaches to the clinic and make it available to all cancer patients so that a larger group of patients and broader cancer types, especially those that do not respond to other therapies could be treated.

In conclusion, engineering approaches for studying tumor microenvironment, including the immune environment, ex vivo provide a great tool for examining drug candidates and help with study of molecular mechanisms of drug action. These approaches could greatly help the clinical trials by providing a means to identify biomarkers of drug responsiveness, efficacy, and toxicity. Furthermore, development of clinically relevant PK/PD models combined with ex vivo experiments can help identify optimal drug combinations as well as timing and dose of drug administration to achieve desired efficacy [83]. Engineering approaches for studying tumor microenvironment can lead to development of ex vivo drug screening tools to provide customized treatment plans for individual patients.

References

1. Turley SJ, Cremasco V, Astarita JL (2015) Immunological hallmarks of stromal cells in the tumour microenvironment. Nat Rev Immunol 15:669–682
2. Adotevi O, Pere H, Ravel P, Haicheur N, Badoual C, Merillon N, Medioni J, Peyrard S, Roncelin S, Verkarre V, Mejean A, Fridman WH, Oudard S, Tartour E (2010) A decrease of regulatory T cells correlates with overall survival after sunitinib-based antiangiogenic therapy in metastatic renal cancer patients. J Immunother 33:991–998
3. Ko JS, Zea AH, Rini BI, Ireland JL, Elson P, Cohen P, Golshayan A, Rayman PA, Wood L, Garcia J, Dreicer R, Bukowski R, Finke JH (2009) Sunitinib mediates reversal of myeloid-derived suppressor cell accumulation in renal cell carcinoma patients. Clin Cancer Res 15:2148–2157
4. Mueller MM, Fusenig NE (2004) Friends or foes – bipolar effects of the tumour stroma in cancer. Nat Rev Cancer 4:839–849
5. Joyce JA, Pollard JW (2009) Microenvironmental regulation of metastasis. Nat Rev Cancer 9:239–252
6. Nakasone ES, Askautrud HA, Kees T, Park JH, Plaks V, Ewald AJ, Fein M, Rasch MG, Tan YX, Qiu J, Park J, Sinha P, Bissell MJ, Frengen E, Werb Z, Egeblad M (2012) Imaging tumor-stroma interactions during chemotherapy reveals contributions of the microenvironment to resistance. Cancer Cell 21:488–503
7. Polyak K, Haviv I, Campbell IG (2009) Co-evolution of tumor cells and their microenvironment. Trends Genet 25:30–38
8. Chen DS, Mellman I (2013) Oncology meets immunology: the cancer-immunity cycle. Immunity 39:1–10
9. Pivarcsi A, Muller A, Hippe A, Rieker J, van Lierop A, Steinhoff M, Seeliger S, Kubitza R, Pippirs U, Meller S, Gerber PA, Liersch R, Buenemann E, Sonkoly E, Wiesner U, Hoffmann TK, Schneider L, Piekorz R, Enderlein E, Reifenberger J, Rohr UP, Haas R, Boukamp P, Haase I, Nurnberg B, Ruzicka T, Zlotnik A, Homey B (2007) Tumor immune escape by the loss of homeostatic chemokine expression. Proc Natl Acad Sci U S A 104:19055–19060
10. Herbst RS, Soria J-C, Kowanetz M, Fine GD, Hamid O, Gordon MS, Sosman JA, McDermott DF, Powderly JD, Gettinger SN, Kohrt HEK, Horn L, Lawrence DP, Rost S, Leabman M, Xiao Y, Mokatrin A, Koeppen H, Hegde PS, Mellman I, Chen DS, Hodi FS (2014) Predictive correlates of response to the anti-PD-L1 antibody MPDL3280A in cancer patients. Nature 515(7528):563–567
11. Powles T, Eder JP, Fine GD, Braiteh FS, Loriot Y, Cruz C, Bellmunt J, Burris HA, Petrylak DP, S-l T, Shen X, Boyd Z, Hegde PS, Chen DS, Vogelzang NJ (2014) MPDL3280A (anti-PD-L1) treatment leads to clinical activity in metastatic bladder cancer. Nature 515(7528):558–562
12. Tumeh PC, Harview CL, Yearley JH, Shintaku IP, Taylor EJM, Robert L, Chmielowski B, Spasic M, Henry G, Ciobanu V, West AN, Carmona M, Kivork C, Seja E, Cherry G, Gutierrez AJ, Grogan TR, Mateus C, Tomasic G, Glaspy JA, Emerson RO, Robins H, Pierce RH, Elashoff DA, Robert C, Ribas A (2014) PD-1 blockade induces responses by inhibiting adaptive immune resistance. Nature 515(7528):568–571
13. Butler TP, Grantham FH, Gullino PM (1975) Bulk transfer of fluid in the interstitial compartment of mammary tumors. Cancer Res 35:3084–3088
14. Fukumura D, Jain RK (2007) Tumor microenvironment abnormalities: causes, consequences, and strategies to normalize. J Cell Biochem 101:937–949

15. Swartz MA, Lund AW (2012) Lymphatic and interstitial flow in the tumour microenviron-ment: linking mechanobiology with immunity. Nat Rev Cancer 12:210–219
16. Hanahan D, Weinberg RA (2011) Hallmarks of cancer: the next generation. Cell 144:646–674
17. DuFort CC, Paszek MJ, Weaver VM (2011) Balancing forces: architectural control of mecha-notransduction. Nat Rev Mol Cell Biol 12:308–319
18. Xu R, Boudreau A, Bissell MJ (2009) Tissue architecture and function: dynamic reciprocity via extra- and intra-cellular matrices. Cancer Metastasis Rev 28:167–176
19. Heldin CH, Rubin K, Pietras K, Ostman A (2004) High interstitial fluid pressure – an obstacle in cancer therapy. Nat Rev Cancer 4:806–813
20. Wiig H (1990) Evaluation of methodologies for measurement of interstitial fluid pressure (Pi): physiological implications of recent Pi data. Crit Rev Biomed Eng 18:27–54
21. Jain RK (2008) Lessons from multidisciplinary translational trials on anti-angiogenic therapy of cancer. Nat Rev Cancer 8:309–316
22. Flessner MF, Choi J, Credit K, Deverkadra R, Henderson K (2005) Resistance of tumor inter-stitial pressure to the penetration of intraperitoneally delivered antibodies into metastatic ovar-ian tumors. Clin Cancer Res 11:3117–3125
23. Wiig H, Tveit E, Hultborn R, Reed RK, Weiss L (1982) Interstitial fluid pressure in DMBA-induced rat mammary tumours. Scand J Clin Lab Invest 42:159–164
24. Raju B, Haug SR, Ibrahim SO, Heyeraas KJ (2008) High interstitial fluid pressure in rat tongue cancer is related to increased lymph vessel area, tumor size, invasiveness and decreased body weight. J Oral Pathol Med 37:137–144
25. Pedersen JA, Boschetti F, Swartz MA (2007) Effects of extracellular fiber architecture on cell membrane shear stress in a 3D fibrous matrix. J Biomech 40:1484–1492
26. Albini A, Sporn MB (2007) The tumour microenvironment as a target for chemoprevention. Nat Rev Cancer 7:139–147
27. Fang X, Sittadjody S, Gyabaah K, Opara EC, Balaji KC (2013) Novel 3D co-culture model for epithelial-stromal cells interaction in prostate cancer. PLoS One 8, e75187
28. Gurski LA, Jha AK, Zhang C, Jia X, Farach-Carson MC (2009) Hyaluronic acid-based hydro-gels as 3D matrices for in vitro evaluation of chemotherapeutic drugs using poorly adherent prostate cancer cells. Biomaterials 30:6076–6085
29. Carvalho MR, Lima D, Reis RL, Correlo VM, Oliveira JM (2015) Evaluating biomaterial- and microfluidic-based 3D tumor models. Trends Biotechnol 33:667–678
30. Cheema U, Brown RA, Alp B, MacRobert AJ (2008) Spatially defined oxygen gradients and vascular endothelial growth factor expression in an engineered 3D cell model. Cell Mol Life Sci 65:177–186
31. Kenny PA, Bissell MJ (2007) Targeting TACE-dependent EGFR ligand shedding in breast cancer. J Clin Invest 117:337–345
32. Ridky TW, Chow JM, Wong DJ, Khavari PA (2010) Invasive three-dimensional organotypic neoplasia from multiple normal human epithelia. Nat Med 16:1450–1455
33. Wozniak MA, Modzelewska K, Kwong L, Keely PJ (2004) Focal adhesion regulation of cell behavior. Biochim Biophys Acta 1692:103–119
34. Rimann M, Graf-Hausner U (2012) Synthetic 3D multicellular systems for drug development. Curr Opin Biotechnol 23:803–809
35. Orlandi P, Barbara C, Bocci G, Fioravanti A, Di Paolo A, Del Tacca M, Danesi R (2005) Idarubicin and idarubicinol effects on breast cancer multicellular spheroids. J Chemother 17:663–667
36. Tung YC, Hsiao AY, Allen SG, Torisawa YS, Ho M, Takayama S (2011) High-throughput 3D spheroid culture and drug testing using a 384 hanging drop array. Analyst 136:473–478
37. Mano JF (2015) Designing biomaterials for tissue engineering based on the deconstruction of the native cellular environment. Mater Lett 141:198–202
38. Goodman TT, Ng CP, Pun SH (2008) 3-D tissue culture systems for the evaluation and optimi-zation of nanoparticle-based drug carriers. Bioconjug Chem 19:1951–1959

39. Li Z, Wang Y, Dong S, Ge C, Xiao Y, Li R, Ma X, Xue Y, Zhang Q, Lv J, Tan Q, Zhu Z, Song X, Tan J (2014) Association of CXCR1 and 2 expressions with gastric cancer metastasis in ex vivo and tumor cell invasion in vitro. Cytokine 69:6–13
40. Rangarajan A, Weinberg RA (2003) Comparative biology of mouse versus human cells: modelling human cancer in mice. Nat Rev Cancer 3:952–959
41. Yamada KM, Cukierman E (2007) Modeling tissue morphogenesis and cancer in 3D. Cell 130:601–610
42. Hwu D, Boutrus S, Greiner C, DiMeo T, Kuperwasser C, Georgakoudi I (2011) Assessment of the role of circulating breast cancer cells in tumor formation and metastatic potential using in vivo flow cytometry. J Biomed Opt 16:040501
43. Sahai E (2007) Illuminating the metastatic process. Nat Rev Cancer 7:737–749
44. Wyckoff JB, Wang Y, Lin EY, Li JF, Goswami S, Stanley ER, Segall JE, Pollard JW, Condeelis J (2007) Direct visualization of macrophage-assisted tumor cell intravasation in mammary tumors. Cancer Res 67:2649–2656
45. Chambers AF, Groom AC, MacDonald IC (2002) Dissemination and growth of cancer cells in metastatic sites. Nat Rev Cancer 2:563–572
46. Boussommier-Calleja A, Li R, Chen MB, Wong SC, Kamm RD (2016) Microfluidics: a new tool for modeling cancer-immune interactions. Trends Cancer 2:6–19
47. Jeon JS, Zervantonakis IK, Chung S, Kamm RD, Charest JL (2013) In vitro model of tumor cell extravasation. PLoS One 8, e56910
48. Lee H, Park W, Ryu H, Jeon NL (2014) A microfluidic platform for quantitative analysis of cancer angiogenesis and intravasation. Biomicrofluidics 8:054102
49. Riahi R, Yang YL, Kim H, Jiang L, Wong PK, Zohar Y (2014) A microfluidic model for organ-specific extravasation of circulating tumor cells. Biomicrofluidics 8:024103
50. Zervantonakis IK, Hughes-Alford SK, Charest JL, Condeelis JS, Gertler FB, Kamm RD (2012) Three-dimensional microfluidic model for tumor cell intravasation and endothelial barrier function. Proc Natl Acad Sci U S A 109:13515–13520
51. Zhang Q, Liu T, Qin J (2012) A microfluidic-based device for study of transendothelial invasion of tumor aggregates in realtime. Lab Chip 12:2837–2842
52. Shin MK, Kim SK, Jung H (2011) Integration of intra- and extravasation in one cell-based microfluidic chip for the study of cancer metastasis. Lab Chip 11:3880–3887
53. Song JW, Cavnar SP, Walker AC, Luker KE, Gupta M, Tung YC, Luker GD, Takayama S (2009) Microfluidic endothelium for studying the intravascular adhesion of metastatic breast cancer cells. PLoS One 4, e5756
54. Kim S, Lee H, Chung M, Jeon NL (2013) Engineering of functional, perfusable 3D microvascular networks on a chip. Lab Chip 13:1489–1500
55. Whisler JA, Chen MB, Kamm RD (2014) Control of perfusable microvascular network morphology using a multiculture microfluidic system. *Tissue engineering Part C*. Methods 20:543–552
56. Jeon JS, Bersini S, Whisler JA, Chen MB, Dubini G, Charest JL, Moretti M, Kamm RD (2014) Generation of 3D functional microvascular networks with human mesenchymal stem cells in microfluidic systems. Integr Biol 6:555–563
57. Chen MB, Whisler JA, Jeon JS, Kamm RD (2013) Mechanisms of tumor cell extravasation in an in vitro microvascular network platform. Integr Biol 5:1262–1271
58. Ehsan SM, Welch-Reardon KM, Waterman ML, Hughes CC, George SC (2014) A three-dimensional in vitro model of tumor cell intravasation. Integr Biol 6:603–610
59. Ghajar CM, Peinado H, Mori H, Matei IR, Evason KJ, Brazier H, Almeida D, Koller A, Hajjar KA, Stainier DY, Chen EI, Lyden D, Bissell MJ (2013) The perivascular niche regulates breast tumour dormancy. Nat Cell Biol 15:807–817
60. Kuo CT, Chiang CL, Chang CH, Liu HK, Huang GS, Huang RY, Lee H, Huang CS, Wo AM (2014) Modeling of cancer metastasis and drug resistance via biomimetic nano-cilia and microfluidics. Biomaterials 35:1562–1571
61. Kuo CT, Liu HK, Huang GS, Chang CH, Chen CL, Chen KC, Huang RY, Lin CH, Lee H, Huang CS, Wo AM (2014) A spatiotemporally defined in vitro microenvironment for controllable signal delivery and drug screening. Analyst 139:4846–4854

62. Bischel LL, Beebe DJ, Sung KE (2015) Microfluidic model of ductal carcinoma in situ with 3D, organotypic structure. BMC Cancer 15:12
63. Sung KE, Yang N, Pehlke C, Keely PJ, Eliceiri KW, Friedl A, Beebe DJ (2011) Transition to invasion in breast cancer: a microfluidic in vitro model enables examination of spatial and temporal effects. Integr Biol 3:439–450
64. Acosta MA, Jiang X, Huang PK, Cutler KB, Grant CS, Walker GM, Gamcsik MP (2014) A microfluidic device to study cancer metastasis under chronic and intermittent hypoxia. Biomicrofluidics 8:054117
65. Pisano M, Triacca V, Barbee KA, Swartz MA (2015) An in vitro model of the tumor-lymphatic microenvironment with simultaneous transendothelial and luminal flows reveals mechanisms of flow enhanced invasion. Integr Biol 7:525–533
66. Kim J, Bae S, An S, Park JK, Kim EM, Hwang SG, Kim WJ, Um HD (2014) Cooperative actions of p21WAF1 and p53 induce Slug protein degradation and suppress cell invasion. EMBO Rep 15:1062–1068
67. Bersini S, Jeon JS, Dubini G, Arrigoni C, Chung S, Charest JL, Moretti M, Kamm RD (2014) A microfluidic 3D in vitro model for specificity of breast cancer metastasis to bone. Biomaterials 35:2454–2461
68. Chaw KC, Manimaran M, Tay EH, Swaminathan S (2007) Multi-step microfluidic device for studying cancer metastasis. Lab Chip 7:1041–1047
69. Bersini S, Jeon JS, Moretti M, Kamm RD (2014) In vitro models of the metastatic cascade: from local invasion to extravasation. Drug Discov Today 19:735–742
70. Fidler IJ (2003) The pathogenesis of cancer metastasis: the 'seed and soil' hypothesis revisited. Nat Rev Cancer 3:453–458
71. Fitzgerald DP, Palmieri D, Hua E, Hargrave E, Herring JM, Qian Y, Vega-Valle E, Weil RJ, Stark AM, Vortmeyer AO, Steeg PS (2008) Reactive glia are recruited by highly proliferative brain metastases of breast cancer and promote tumor cell colonization. Clin Exp Metastasis 25:799–810
72. Huh D, Matthews BD, Mammoto A, Montoya-Zavala M, Hsin HY, Ingber DE (2010) Reconstituting organ-level lung functions on a chip. Science 328:1662–1668
73. Aref RA, Huang RJ, Weimian Y, Weng S, Thiery JP, Kamm RD (2013) Screening therapeutic EMT blocking agents. Integr Biol 5:381–389
74. Zhu Z, Aref AR et al (2014) Inhibition of KRAS-driven tumorigenicity by interruption of an autocrine cytokine circuit. Cancer Discov 4:452–465
75. Barbie TU, Alexe G, Zhu Z, Aref AR, Hahn WC, Barbie DA, Gillanders WE (2014) IKKε induces a cytokine signaling network essential for tumorigenicity. J Clin Invest 124(12):5411–5423
76. Hirt C, Papadimitropoulos A, Mele V, Muraro MG, Mengus C, Iezzi G, Terracciano L, Martin I, Spagnoli GC (2014) "In vitro" 3D models of tumor-immune system interaction. Adv Drug Deliv Rev 79–80:145–154
77. Tan L et al (2014) Overcoming FGFR-resistance with covalent inhibitors. Proc Natl Acad Sci U S A 109:11–45. Li Tan, Jun Wang, Junko Tanizaki, Zhifeng Huang, Amir R. Aref, Maria Rusan, Su-Jie Zhu, Yiyun Zhang, Dalia Ercan, Rachel G. Liao, Marzia Capelletti, Wenjun Zhou, Wooyoung Hur, NamDoo Kim, Taebo Sim, Suzanne Gaudet, David A. Barbie, Jing-Ruey Joanna Yeh, Cai-Hong Yun, Peter S. Hammerman, Moosa Mohammadi, Pasi A. Jänne, and Nathanael S. Gray Development of covalent inhibitors that can overcome resistance to first-generation FGFR kinase inhibitors PNAS 2014 111 (45) E4869–E4877; published ahead of print October 27, 2014, doi:10.1073/pnas.1403438111.
78. Swartz MA, Hirosue S, Hubbell JA (2012) Engineering approaches to immunotherapy. Sci Transl Med 4:148–149
79. Hamid O, Robert C, Daud A, Hodi FS, Hwu W-J, Kefford R, Wolchok JD, Hersey P, Joseph RW, Weber JS, Dronca R, Gangadhar TC, Patnaik A, Zarour H, Joshua AM, Gergich K, Elassaiss-Schaap J, Algazi A, Mateus C, Boasberg P, Tumeh PC, Chmielowski B, Ebbinghaus SW, Li XN, Kang SP and Ribas A. N Engl J Med. 2013 Jul 11;369(2):134-44. doi:10.1056/NEJMoa1305133. Epub 2013 Jun 2.Safety and tumor responses with lambrolizumab (anti-PD-1) in melanoma.

80. Wolchok JD, Kluger H, Callahan MK, Postow MA, Rizvi NA, Lesokhin AM, Segal NH, Ariyan CE, Gordon R-A, Reed K, Burke MM, Caldwell A, Kronenberg SA, Agunwamba BU, Zhang X, Lowy I, Inzunza HD, Feely W, Horak CE, Hong Q, Korman AJ, Wigginton JM, Gupta A and Sznol M. N Engl J Med. 2013 Jul 11;369(2):122–33. doi:10.1056/NEJMoa1302369. Epub 2013 Jun 2.Nivolumab plus ipilimumab in advanced melanoma.
81. Sharma P and Allison JP (2015) Immune checkpoint targeting in cancer therapy: toward combination strategies with curative potential. Cell. 161(2):205–14. doi:10.1016/j.cell.2015.03.030.
82. Turcotte S, Rosenberg SA (2011) Immunotherapy for metastatic solid cancers. Adv Surg 45:341–360
83. Bhatia SN, Ingber DE (2014) Microfluidic organs-on-chips. Nat Biotechnol 32:760–772

Advancing Techniques and Insights in Circulating Tumor Cell (CTC) Research

Bee Luan Khoo*, Parthiv Kant Chaudhuri*, Chwee Teck Lim, and Majid Ebrahimi Warkiani

1 Introduction

Cancer is a major cause of mortality worldwide, with a disease burden estimated to grow over the coming decades. Circulating tumor cells (CTCs) are rare cancer cells released from the primary or metastatic tumors and transported though the peripheral circulatory system to their specific secondary locations. The presence of CTCs in a cancer patient's blood has been used as a prognostic biomarker, with lower CTC count correlating with greater overall survival [1]. In spite of its clinical potential, the isolation and detection of CTCs has been a challenging task due to its rare presence amongst other blood cells (as low as 1–10 CTCs per billions of blood cells) and variability in terms of both morphological and biochemical markers. Recent developments of microfluidics technology have paved the way for better isolation and characterization of CTCs due to several advantages such as lower sample volume, higher sensitivity and throughput and lesser production cost [2, 3].

*Author contributed equally with all other contributors.

B.L. Khoo
BioSystems and Micromechanics (BioSyM) IRG, Singapore-MIT Alliance for Research and Technology (SMART) Centre, Singapore

P.K. Chaudhuri
Mechanobiology Institute, National University of Singapore, Singapore

C.T. Lim
Mechanobiology Institute, National University of Singapore, SINGAPORE and Department of Biomedical Engineering, National University of Singapore, Singapore

M.E. Warkiani (✉)
School of Mechanical and Manufacturing Engineering, Australian Centre for NanoMedicine, Garvan Institute for Biomedical Research, University of New South Wales, Sydney, Australia

School of Medical Sciences, Edith Cowan University, Perth, Australia
e-mail: m.warkiani@unsw.edu.au

© Springer International Publishing Switzerland 2017
A.R. Aref, D. Barbie (eds.), *Ex Vivo Engineering of the Tumor Microenvironment*, Cancer Drug Discovery and Development, DOI 10.1007/978-3-319-45397-2_5

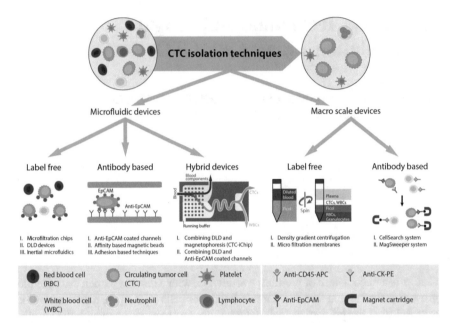

Fig. 1 Schematic classifications of various circulating tumor cell (CTC) isolation technologies. CTC isolation platforms can be classified into two major classes: microfluidics and conventional macro scale devices. The microfluidic devices can be further sub-divided into label-free (microfiltration, deterministic lateral displacement (DLD) devices and inertial microfluidics), antibody-based (anti-EpCAM coated channels, affinity-based magnetic beads and adhesion-based techniques) and hybrid techniques (combining DLD with magnetophoresis or anti-EpCAM coated channels) that uses the advantages of both label-free and antibody-based methods. Macro scale techniques can also be further classified into label-free (density gradient centrifugation and micro filtration membranes) and antibody-based (CellSearch system, MagSweeper system) platforms

In this chapter, various CTC isolation devices are classified under two major categories: microfluidics and conventional macro-scale devices, as illustrated in Fig. 1. We will be discussing both label-free methods and antibody-dependent methods for CTC isolation, and will provide discussion and future perspectives on the advantages and drawbacks of both these techniques on potential clinical applications. Advancement in these technologies for CTCs and associated components, such as exosomes, led to an unraveling of tumor variation, ranging histology, molecular, proteomic and functional heterogeneity, which will be discussed in the subsequent sections.

CTCs are heterogeneous in terms of the morphology and surface expression of various biomarkers. Therefore, it is an uphill task to isolate these rare cells from clinical samples in the presence of billions of other hematologic cells. Recent technological advancements observed that CTCs differ from blood cells in various biophysical properties (such as size, adhesion and stiffness) and cell surface receptor expressions (such as Epithelial cell adhesion molecule (EpCAM) and Cytokeratin (CK)) [4, 5]. Current microfluidics techniques and conventional methods can target such distinct properties of the CTCs and achieve high isolation efficiency and throughput along with greater cell viability for downstream single-cell analysis.

2 Microfluidics Devices

Over the past decade, microfluidics technologies have been extensively utilized for study of human disease such as cancer. Microfluidic systems normally leverage on the disparities in the intrinsic properties of the different cell populations (i.e., size, deformability, surface charge, density, etc.) to achieve separations. Isolation and characterization of CTCs using microfluidic systems has been a flourishing area of research which can be broadly categorized to label-free and antibody-based approaches (see Fig. 1).

2.1 Label-Free Technologies

Differences in the biophysical properties between the CTCs and blood cells, such as size, deformability, magnetic susceptibility and electrical behaviors have been exploited to develop label-free sorting of CTCs. The key advantages of this method compared to the antibody-based devices are the collection of a complete pool of CTC population consisting of both EpCAM positive and negative cells and greater compatibility to a wide range of assays that require viable unlabeled cells. Size and deformability-based sorting of CTCs can be achieved by using microfiltration devices and a membrane pore size of around 8 μm has been proved optimal for CTCs capturing [6]. The size of the CTCs varies between 6 and 30 μm and is usually greater than normal hematologic cells [7]. 3D membrane micro filter consisting of two-layers of membrane has been developed with the upper membrane pore size diameter of 9 μm and the pores are aligned centrally to the smaller pores (8 μm) on the basal layer [8]. When blood samples are passed through the device, the CTCs are captured in the upper membrane while other blood cells pass through the gap between the two membranes. This device has an isolation efficiency of 86 % and processing throughput of 3.75 ml/min. Recently, a novel design of the 3D membrane micro filter is introduced with 5 times greater upper membrane pore diameter than that of the lower membrane pores (8 μm) [9]. The CTCs are captured between the gap of the two membranes and the cell can be analyzed by separating the two membranes. Isolation efficiency ranging from 78 to 83 % can be obtained using this device with higher cell viability (greater than 70 %). In order to mitigate the pressure buildup problem during membrane filtration, cross-flow conformation in parallel direction to the filtration membrane was introduced [10]. Membrane microfilters developed using this principle can obtain a capture efficiency of 98 % for MCF-7 cells spiked into blood samples. In another interesting study, weir-shaped structures are used as barrier across the filtration chip to trap most of the CTCs while the blood cells can pass through the narrow opening at the upper portion of the barrier [11]. This device has an isolation efficiency of >95 % and processing speed of 20 ml/h. Microfiltration devices can also be integrated with conical shaped holes to achieve highly efficient cell capture (96 %) at 0.2 ml/min processing rate, as illustrated in

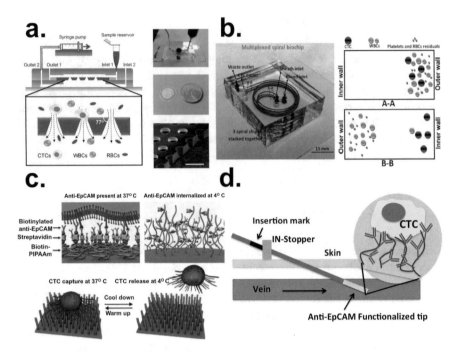

Fig. 2 Diagrammatic representation of CTC isolation devices. (**a**) Integration of microfiltration with conical holes for size-based capturing of CTCs. The sample is processed through inlet 1 and it passes through the filter and subsequently gets collected by constant pulling from a syringe pump at outlet 2 (*top right*). Representation of the microfluidics platform processing clinical samples (*middle right*). Image of 9 mm diameter micro-filter (*bottom right*). Scanning electron micrograph (SEM) of conical holes (scale 40 μm). Reproduced with permission from [10]. (**b**) Representation of multiplexed spiral biochip with two inlets for clinical samples and sheath fluid respectively. The CTCs are sorted due to the action of inertial lift and Dean drag forces and are segregated towards the inner wall of the microfluidics channel (A–A) whereas the WBCs and platelets are concentrated towards the outer wall (B–B). Reproduced with permission from [12]. (**c**) Working principle of Thermoresponsive NanoVelcro substrate for capturing CTCs with biotinylated anti-EpCAM antibodies at 37 °C and subsequent release of the captured CTCs at 4 °C due to temperature-dependent conformational changes of the polymer brushes that changes the availability of anti-EpCAM antibodies on the surface. Reproduced with permission from [13]. (**d**) Schematic of the working principle of Gilupi nanodetector system for capturing CTCs from the in-vivo environment. The gold-plated medical steel wire is coated with hydrogel (indicated in *brown*) and functionalized with anti-EpCAM antibodies (indicated in *red*) and is inserted into the patient vein to capture EpCAM positive CTCs. Reproduced with permission from [14] (Color figure online)

Fig. 2a [10]. Clearbridge Biomedics has commercialized a microfluidics device, the CTChip® with an array of crescent-shaped structures composed of three closely spaced micropillars that can trap the CTCs from clinical samples with high throughput and without channel clogging from the cell debris [15, 16]. This device can isolate single and double CTCs and the viable cells can be retrieved and cultured by reversing the flow direction. ISET® (Rarecells, Paris, France) and ScreenCell® are two commercialized systems for sized-based isolation of CTCs that provide cost-effective and high-throughput enrichment of fixed and viable CTCs respectively [17, 18]. The major advantages of the microfiltration devices are its simple design and its ability to obtain the CTCs from the whole blood in a single pass while maintaining its cellular integrity for detection and further downstream analysis. Although size based enrichment of CTCs provides a high-throughput, label-free technique, it has some drawbacks; such as the cells are subjected to high mechanical stress that can alter their normal function [19] and there is a size overlap between the CTCs and leukocytes that can increase the probability of isolating more contaminating cells [20].

Dielectrophoresis (DEP) phenomena have also been used for CTC isolation based on the differential motion of the cells when exposed to a non-uniform electric field. Cells can exhibit attractive and repulsive behaviors depending on their size and dielectric polarizability under a non-uniform electric field [21]. Compared to normal cells, CTCs have greater surface area and higher capacitance per unit area that provides them a unique dielectric property and thereby affecting their motion in presence of an electric field. Contactless DEP (cDEP) is developed with greater sensitivity and eliminating the drawbacks of traditional DEP such as high cost, air bubble production, electrode delamination and culture contamination [22]. This device reports an isolation efficiency of 64.5 % for carcinoma cells from concentrated RBC solution. ApoCell laboratories have commercialized ApoStream device in 2010 and validation study using breast cancer cells spiked into clinical sample has observed an isolation efficiency of 86.6 % with higher viability (97.6 %) [23]. The main advantage of DEP devices is that the effect of therapeutic agents could be determined by monitoring the differences in the frequency responses of the cells under the action of various chemotherapeutic agents.

Deterministic lateral displacement (DLD) is another label-free method used for sorting CTCs in microfluidic devices. A novel DLD platform with 58 μm triangular micropost and 42 μm gap is used to capture CTCs at high efficiency (>85 %) and throughput (10 ml/min) [24]. Inertial microfluidics is also used for isolating CTCs by combining inertial lift forces and pinched flow dynamics to focus particles in their preferential equilibrium position along a microfluidic channel. Inertial microfluidics can be combined with microvortex particle capturing to isolate CTCs in a high-throughput, clogging free manner [25]. Apart from straight channels, spiral microfluidics can be used to achieve inertial sorting by combining inertial and Dean drag forces. Our group developed a spiral microfluidics chip with rectangular cross section to isolate CTCs (varying from 5 to 88 CTCs/ml of blood) from 20 metastatic lung cancer patients [26]. Strong inertial lift forces focus the bigger CTCs towards the inner wall while the smaller hematologic cells move towards the outer wall. Due to greater channel dimensions (500 μm width and 160 μm height) and increased flow rate (3 ml/h), clogging of the microchannels by the cell debris is also mitigated, thereby increasing the performance and sensitivity of the device. More recently, we further developed our spiral microfluidics chip with trapezoidal cross-section that can separate the CTCs from metastatic breast and lung cancer clinical samples in an ultra-high throughput manner (7.5 ml within 8 min) [27]. Our group subsequently developed multiplexed spiral microfluidics chip for ultra-high throughput sorting of viable clinical CTC (12–1275 CTCs/ml for breast cancer patients and 10–1535 CTCs/ml for lung cancer patients) for further downstream single-cell characterization such as fluorescence in-situ hybridization (FISH) and proteomics analysis, as represented in Fig. 2b [12]. In another study, contraction-expansion array microfluidic channels is used to enrich cancer cells spiked into blood suspension with 99.5 % efficiency [28]. In negative selection methods, the CTCs are untouched; however the RBCs are lysed and the WBCs are magnetically removed using specific markers such as CD45, CD61 [29].

2.2 Antibody Based Technologies

Antibody mediated CTC isolation techniques are dependent on the specific binding of the cell surface receptors with the antibody bound matrix. The matrix could be of mainly two types, such as magnetic beads or functionalized microfluidics channel. The two commonly used markers for CTC isolation and detection are EpCAM and different subtype of CK. However, due to the occurrence of epithelial to mesenchymal transition (EMT), all CTCs do not express these markers and therefore these techniques fail to collect some subpopulations of the CTCs [30, 31]. CTCs can be selectively labeled with antibody-tagged magnetic microbeads (diameter: 0.5–5 μm) or nanoparticles (diameter: 50–250 nm) and sorted in a non-uniform magnetic field, whereby the labeled CTCs migrate to a region of higher magnetic field and get trapped with an isolation efficiency of 86 % [32, 33]. A straight microchannel with many square indentation on its sidewalls can be used to pull and trap the EpCAM tagged CTCs towards the sidewalls under the influence of an external magnetic field [34]. Fluxion Biosciences have commercialized a microfluidics device, IsoFlux™, which can trap magnetically labeled CTCs when passed through a microchannel with uniform magnetic field. Other promising strategies to further develop the enrichment of EpCAM-positive CTCs in a highly sensitive and efficient manner includes 3D nanostructured substrate or nano "Fly Paper" Technology [35] and a Velcro-like microfluidics platform with isolation efficiency ranging from 40 to 70 %, as depicted in Fig. 2c [13].

Adhesion-based CTC isolation techniques depend on the binding affinity of CTCs to a surface whose biochemical (using antibody coated surface) and structural properties (using nano topographical features) can be modified to favor suitable adhesion. This technique can be performed either in static [36] or dynamic flow modes [37], while the later one is more sensitive due to the greater interaction between the cells and the surface and prevention of non-specific adhesion due to fluid shear forces. Using 3D structures such as microposts inside a microfluidics channel (the CTC-Chip), the effective surface area can be enhanced and the collision frequency between the cell and the EpCAM functionalized surface can be increased [38]. The CTC-Chip has recovery rate of 60 % and the recovery efficiency does not depend on the different expression of EpCAM by the CTCs due to the greater collision frequency. Geometrically enhanced differential immunocapture

(GEDI) chip is developed to further increase the effective collision frequency between the CTCs and the antibody-coated microstructure to enhance the isolation efficiency (~90%) [37]. In another study, herringbone-chip was discovered with anti-EpCAM coated herringbones structures to increase the collision between the CTCs and antibody functionalized PDMS channels [39]. This device has an isolation efficiency of 91.8% with 95% cell viability. Recently, geometrically enhanced mixing (GEM) chip is introduced with a further improved herringbone micromixers to enhance the throughput and isolation purity in antibody-dependent devices [40]. CTCs are detected using this device in 17 out of the 18 pancreatic cancer patients studied and the CTC number correlates with the tumor size in three advanced stage patients during the period of the treatment. Adhesion-based CTC isolation techniques using micropost arrays has been commercialized by OnQChip™ (On-Q-ity, MA, USA) and the CEE™ chip (Biocept Laboratories, CA, USA). Graphene oxide sheets can be functionalized with anti-EpCAM antibodies and adsorbed on gold patterned substrates for efficient and sensitive enrichment of CTCs [41]. The increased surface area and biocompatibility of graphene oxide enables greater loading capacity of anti-EpCAM antibodies on its surface and the isolated cells can be cultured on the gold substrates for further downstream characterization such as RT-PCR and drug testing.

Different techniques can be combined to create a better hybrid platform for effective enrichment of CTCs with higher throughput. The CTC-iChip uses both antigen dependent (magnetophoresis) and independent (DLD with inertial focusing) strategies to isolate CTCs with greater sensitive (0.5 CTCs per ml) from clinical samples with lower CTC numbers [42]. Another study combined DLD with EpCAM functionalized isolation chambers to enrich CTCs with greater efficiency (90%) and throughput (9.6 ml/min) [43]. CTCs are initially sorted from other blood cells in the DLD compartment comprising of triangular microposts and subsequently they are captured in an EpCAM functionalized chambers with fishbone conformation to enhance the isolation capacity.

3   Conventional Macro Scale Devices

3.1   Label-Free Technologies

Density gradient centrifugation is a label-free technique using centrifugal forces for sorting cells from blood based on the difference in their sedimentation coefficient. When a clinical sample is subjected to density gradient centrifugation, the denser RBC and neutrophils settles at the base of the tube whereas the CTCs, plasma and mononucleated cells are collected above the buffy coat. In another study using silicon-blending oil as a floatation media, cancer cells are identified in 53% and 33% of gastrointestinal tract cancer and breast cancer patients respectively [44]. OncoQuick centrifugation system has been developed with a porous membrane within the centrifugation tube to prevent the mixing of the separation media with the clinical sample before centrifugation. This system has a greater CTC isolation efficiency compared to the Ficoll density gradient centrifugation [45]. OncoQuick has been used for the enrichment of CTCs from metastatic breast cancer patients and it can successfully detect CTCs in 69.2 % of the clinical samples [46]. RBCs and WBCs can be cross-linked to form rosettes using a cocktail of antibodies and RosetteSep™ (STEMCELL Tech., BC, Canada) commercialized this technique. On application of centrifugal forces these rosettes can be efficiently separated from the CTCs due to their greater densities [47]. In another study, the use of sieve material as a filter with pore size of 4.5 μm could separate 100 % of the HeLa cells spiked into blood and detect cancer cells in 19 out of the 50 cancer patient specimen [48].

3.2 Antibody Based Technologies

Notable achievement in the isolation techniques of CTCs has been accomplished by the introduction of FDA (Food and Drug Administration)–approved method, the CellSearch system (Veridex) [49, 50]. CellSearch system consists of a semi-automated platform for capturing EpCAM positive CTCs using immunomagnetic cell sorting and the cells are subsequently identified by antibody staining of various subtypes of cytokeratins. This system was validated for CTC detection in metastatic breast cancer patients and it was reported that CTC assessment could provide critical prognostic information such as overall survival and progression-free survival [51–53]. However, CellSearch system can only successfully isolate EpCAM positive sub-population of the CTCs and the isolated CTCs are permanently labeled with antibodies that limit their downstream characterization. Illumina Inc. (CA, USA) commercialized MagSweeper system, which consists of a robotic arm with a magnetic rod that continuously shifts the region of high magnetic field within a multiwell plate [54]. The speed and trajectory of the rod movement has been standardized to favor the adsorption of EpCAM-labeled CTCs on the rod and prevents non-specific adsorption by other non-target cells. This system can perform at a high throughput (9 ml/h) and higher isolation efficiency (~81 %). Flow cytometry technologies such as fluorescence-activated cell sorting (FACS) can be utilized to simultaneously detect several fluorescently labeled antibodies and thereby increasing CTC isolation purity [55]. However, this technique can not provide greater sensitivity for CTC isolation due to the varied expression pattern of different antigens on the CTCs depending on the types and stages of cancer [56]. Anti-EpCAM coated detachable microbeads can be used to enlarge the size of the CTCs before passaging the whole blood sample through the microfiltration device (8 μm pore size) [57]. Leukocytes and other blood cells can pass through the filter while the larger CTCs remain trapped on the filter membrane. This device reports a capture efficiency of 89 % and isolated 1–31 CTCs/ml of clinical samples. CTCs can also be isolated directly from the in vivo environment using the Gilupi nanodetector®

system, as shown in Fig. 2D [14]. The nanodetector is coated with anti-EpCAM antibodies and inserted in the peripheral arm vein for 30 min to collect larger number of CTCs.

4   Characterization of Cancer Cell Heterogeneity

Tumors demonstrate huge heterogeneity in morphology, immuno-phenotype, and genotype [58]. Novel therapeutic approaches for BRAF mutant cutaneous melanoma [59] and ALK rearranged NSCLC [60], in the recent decades have been unable to increase the survival of patients with advanced stage cancer. This is largely attributed to tumor heterogeneity and the rise of drug tolerant or resistant subtypes under the influence of ineffective drug therapy [61]. Similarly, CTCs have been found to demonstrate a similar range of heterogeneity across multiple parameters, including morphology, histology and proteomics (Fig. 3).

4.1   Histology and Morphology

Observations of tumor histology are often correlated with disease severity [65], and have been found to exhibit strong correlations to genotype [66]. Generally, malignant cancer cells are identified as cells with a round or oval nucleus, and a high nuclear to cytoplasmic (N/C) ratio [67]. However, cancer subtypes display distinct morphology variations, such as the established case of small cell lung cancer (SCLC) and non-small cell lung cancer (NSCLC) [68].

Recent analysis with specific cancer subpopulations [62, 69, 70], such as disseminated tumor cells (DTCs) and CTCs revealed extensive intertumor histological variation (within the same tumor type among individuals) [71]. CTCs are derived from the blood samples of cancer patients and selectively isolated by targeting protein expression [49], negative selection [29], physical properties [26, 42], or by means of expansion [8, 63, 72]. CTCs can be isolated on a routine basis via a non-invasive process of blood withdrawal [73], allowing monitoring of therapy-associated changes in protein expression, a process which could illuminate the mechanisms that facilitate drug resistance development. Proteomics profiling of CTCs has revealed some of the extent of heterogeneity present. Results suggest the role of multiple pathways, such as the process of EMT transition [74], which is involved in the metastatic cascade [75, 76]. CTC size and other physical parameters may also vary significantly [77], which limits the sensitivity of CTC enrichment devices. These variations can be observed within the cells obtained from tumors of the same patient. Upcoming high throughput spectral imaging techniques will allow rapid processing of single-cell images, providing dynamic insights to cancer cell morphological changes under stimulus or drug exposure (see Fig. 3a) [78, 79].

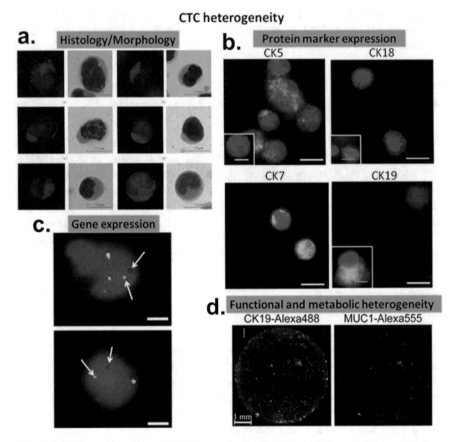

Fig. 3 Varied manifestation of CTC heterogeneity. (**a**) Pleomorphism of CTC morphology obtained from the same patient demonstrated with immunofluorescence staining (*left*) and Papanicolau stain (*right*) [62]. (**b**) Immunostaining of various forms of cytokeratin reveals heterogeneity in protein marker expression. Representative images of minority cohort are provided in boxed images (*bottom left*). Scale bar, 20 μm [63]. (**c**) Molecular FISH analysis carried out with clinical human CTCs from an NSCLC patient using Vysis ALK Break Apart FISH probe. Varied frequency of separation of the original gene fusion signal (*arrows*) is detected in cells obtained from the same sample [12]. Scale bar: 16 mm [12]. (**d**) Antibody coated membranes demonstrates active protein secretion of CK19 (*green*) and MUC1 (*red*) from viable CTCs respectively [64] (Color figure online)

4.2 Proteomics and Genetic Profiling

Although some histology aspects of cancer cells correspond to genotype, intertumor variation in protein expression has been identified in tumors classified under similar subtypes [80]. Depending on the microenvironment [81], as well as tissue organization and composition [82], cancer cells may be exposed to varying stimulus which induces different rates of oncogene or tumor suppressor gene expressions.

For example, accumulation of mutations in the adenomatous polyposis coli (APC) gene may lead to abnormal production of APC protein, an alteration associated with increased colorectal cancer risk [83]. Cancer cells presented with the APC mutation also has increased resistance towards certain drug strategies [84].

The varied protein expression often confers cancer cells with favorable characteristics for growth and survival. For example, the amplified production of human epidermal growth factor receptor 2 (HER2) has been suggested to induce cluster formation in membranes, leading to heightened susceptibility to tumorigenesis [85]. Processing and comparison of large databases have led to resources that provide quantitative values for EMT phenotypes, based on various protein expressions [86]. These dynamics have hindered attempts to completely map the extent of cancer heterogeneity [87]. Our inability to fully comprehend cancer progression often generates conflicting hypotheses and reduces our ability to generate effective treatment strategies.

4.2.1 Understanding CTC Proteomics for Diagnostic and Prognostic Relevance

Tumor-associated proteins have been regularly identified to characterize cancer for administering precise therapeutic treatment. The golden standard involves extraction of these proteins from tumor biopsies [88]. However, few proteins demonstrate actual clinical utility due to cancer heterogeneity [89], except for few instances such as the prostate-specific antigen (PSA). CTC has been broadly defined in a similar way as DTCs [90], namely being positive for epithelial markers (e.g. EpCAM and CKs) and negative for leukocyte markers. However, the proteomics of CTCs are extremely varied (Fig. 3b), and may even not reflect the phenotype observed from the tumor(s) of the same patient. Hence, researchers have been looking for unique specific markers.

To better identify the full CTC spectrum, researchers have started to explore tumour-associated proteins detectable in the serum. Although the field of serum proteomics is in its infancy, technological advances are surfacing which will aid in identifying novel markers. The serum proteome of tumors is a rich source for the analysis of cancer cell activity and interaction with the tumor niche [91]. Circulating tumor DNA (ctDNA), which are short fragments of 150–200 bp DNA, are released from apoptotic CTCs and are now a major interest for diagnostic purposes [92]. ctDNA constitutes about 3–93 % of the total cell-free DNA (cfDNA) and ctDNA can be used as a liquid biopsy biomarker for cancer treatment by analyzing somatic mutations, chromosomal aberrations and loss of heterozygosity [93]. Recently, de novo multiplexed identification of ctDNA mutation is performed from different types of tumor (SHIVA trial) and 28 of 29 mutations detected in the tissue biopsy can be identified in the ctDNA from 27 cancer patients. This signifies the potential of ctDNA as a biomarker [94]. DEP microelectrodes can be used for the isolation of ctDNA from whole blood; however, this system is unsuitable for separation of small fragments of apoptotic DNA (<0.01 μm) and the use of DEP microelectrodes also suffers from cross-sample contamination issues and higher fabrication cost [95, 96].

In another study, digital PCR is used to define malignant growth in various types of cancer such as pancreatic, ovarian, colorectal and they can identify ctDNAs in greater than 75% of the patients [97]. Additionally, next generation sequencing (NGS) techniques has also been used for sequencing ctDNA and to monitor the response of patients to anti-cancer treatments [98]. ctDNA retains the spectrum of gene mutations found in tumours, and has the same ability to capture mutation patterns as per tumor biopsies [94]. A supposed advantage of utilizing ctDNA is the heightened abundance of material over CTCs, as well as the ease of detection over capturing CTCs [97]. Most importantly, the technology advancement in DNA profiling has enabled sensitive detection of a small amount of genetic material, in fact less than the amount of genetic material within a single CTC [93].

MicroRNAs (miRs) are small (20–22 bases), single stranded fragments of nucleic acid that can negatively regulate gene expression and many tumors have a characteristic miR-based tissue profiles. The miRs can be released into the microenvironment due to an active process or via passive secretion from a dying cancer cell; however, some miRs are not secreted from tumor cells [99]. Circulating miRs can be identified from serum and plasma of clinical samples and different types of solid tumors such as breast, colon, gastric can be distinguished based on miR profiles [100]. miRs from cancer cells [101] may also be isolated from plasma or found within microvesicles (100–1000 nm) [102], exosomes [103] and oncosomes (1–10 μm) (Fig. 4). Exosomes are cell-derived nanovesicles (30–100 nm) that are secreted into tumor microenvironment and play a critical role in cell-cell communication. Exosomes contains genetic information and signaling molecules including proteins, lipids, mRNA, miR and dsDNA that help in the formation of the premetastatic niche at the secondary tumor site [104, 105]. Exosomes can be extracted from the body fluids using conventional methods such as ultracentrifugation and combination of sucrose gradient ultracentrifugation with ultrafiltration centrifugation. However, the former method is much simpler in terms of sample preparation (requires 4–5 h) and has greater isolation efficiency (5–25%) [106]. Recently, Exo-Quick™ (System Biosciences) and Exo-spin™ (Cell Guidance System) commercialized the isolation kits for exosomes in a cost effective and user-friendly manner. Exosomes can also be isolated by targeting antibody-immobilized magnetic beads against specific antigens that are expressed on their surface such as Alix, annexin, EpCAM, Rab5, CD63, CD81, CD82, CD9 [107]. This technique has greater isolation efficiency than conventional methods; however, it fails to collect the entire population, as some of the exosomes do not express the targeted protein on its surface. Microfluidics isolation of exosomes has been developed using ExoChip, which uses fluorescent imaging to quantify the exosomes that are captured on anti-CD63 coated chips [108]. Interestingly, this study observed a greater number of exosomes in cancer patients (2.34 ± 0.31 fold higher) compared to healthy individuals, which indicates the significance of exosomes as a circulating biomarker. Microfiltration devices (with membrane pore size of <500 nm) have also been used for exosome sorting from whole blood in a highly efficient manner [109]. This device can be combined with electrophoresis and pressure driven flow to further increase the enrichment efficiency. Label-free identification of exosomes can be

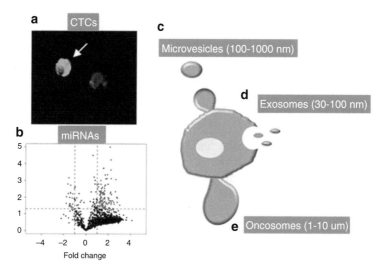

Fig. 4 Utilizing CTC components for diagnostic and prognostic relevance. (**a**) Intact CTCs are the primary targets for isolation and enrichment for further analysis and utility. A representative image of enriched CTCs (*white arrow*) is provided (*Green*: cytokeratin; *Red*: CD45; *Blue*: Nuclei stain, Hoechst). Scale bar: 20 mm [12]. (**b**) An example of a scatter plot demonstrating the differential signal intensities of miRNAs isolated from serum samples of cancer patients and healthy controls [101]. (**c–e**) Extracellular vesicles can be classified into three categories based on size—microvesicles, exosomes and large oncosomes. Oncosomes appear to display unique properties and could serve as an important target for cancer characterization (Color figure online)

carried out using surface plasmon resonance (SPR) sensor chip, the nano-plasmonic exosome (nPLEX) [110]. The nPLEX chip can be functionalized with various exosomal antibodies and can potentially identify 12 exosomal markers within 30 min.

Research for novel markers in glioma has been extensive for the recent years, and several new markers such as CXCR4 [111] and haptoglobin [91] has been discovered. However, the heterogeneity of cancer complicates the validation of any new candidate markers, and extensive single-cell analysis will be required. Some clinicians are also keen to utilize the serum markers from CTCs, namely exosomes and ctDNA, as diagnostic markers for cancer. For example, the mutant EGFRvIII protein, found in exosomes [112], has been demonstrated as a potential therapeutic marker. Markers from ctDNA, such as miR181 [113], can also be a source for diagnostic means, if the half-life of ctDNA is established [114]. To overcome the problem of information loss due to DNA degradation, extracellular vesicles (EVs) may also be extracted from blood serum. EVs are vesicles that bud off from membranes or secreted from cells for intercellular communication [115], and the transported components are protected from degradation. In the latter instance, these vesicles form exosomes [116].

Another alternative to overcoming the low genetic material available from rare cancer cell subpopulations, such as CTCs, is via single-cell analysis (SCA). Advanced systems, such as the microfluidic image cytometry (MIC) [117] and mass cytometry platform (CyTOF) [118], are available. They can simultaneously separate, process and analysis information from large panels of protein expression, such as the Akt kinase [119, 120].

4.3 Molecular Profiling

Ideally, CTCs can help to reflect the complete tumor spectrum, if the technological limitations impeding enrichment and analysis of rare cells are overcome. Recent advances now allow the simultaneous monitoring of multiple gene expression in parallel. Sensitive transcriptomic tools, such as the single-cell PCR based approach (SINCE-PCR) [121], serve to obtain quantitative and qualitative information which can be beneficial in both scientific and clinical settings. Single-cell analysis can also be carried out with fluorescence in-situ hybridization (FISH) (Fig. 3c).

Thus far, the identification of CTCs has been made complicated due to the lack of specificity of known markers. In fact, most existing molecular subtyping methods do not distinguish cancer cells from normal stroma tissue. Varied histopathological sub-types [122] exhibit different sensitivity of markers as well, and some markers may be common across several cancer types [123, 124]. Variation also exists across tumors from the same patient [125, 126], and some specific cancer types only have traces of molecular similarity with other cancer types [127]. This hinders the accuracy of tumor profiling, since the small amount of clinical samples may be insufficient to reveal rare mutations or intrinsic changes that occurred from response to therapeutic treatment [128]. Such extent of tumor heterogeneity may contribute to differential response to anti-cancer treatment [93], due to incomplete tumor profiling or adaptation to evade treatment.

The rise in advanced technologies, such as the Ensemble Decision Aliquot Ranking (eDAR), is now revealing vast heterogeneity in CTC gene expression, both within and across different patients [129]. An integrative approach to enrich, recover and characterize CTC exomes enabled extensive profiling of prostate CTCs. These profiles revealed a match to a portion of the tumor tissue from the same patient [130]. The spectrum of mutations varied significantly from cell lines, highlighting the issue of translational relevance of immortalized cancer cell phenotypes [131]. Extensive profiling also enables mapping of clonality. Preliminary studies suggest that the cells from the original tumor and metastases are phenotypically distinct, but presence of non-metastatic intermediate phenotypes which are found to persist in both the original tumor and its metastases [132]. Screening of various nuclei at the single-cell level also revealed extensive heterogeneity for KRAS, PIK3CA and other gene expressions [133–135]. These molecular variations may be the reason for a high failure in various anti-cancer regimes, due to an inaccurate diagnosis, or because the drugs are unable to target all cancer subtypes [93]. Detailed single-cell profiling of tumors may reveal novel mechanisms of tumor progression, such as gene amplification (e.g. MET) or chromosomal rearrangements [e.g. ALK (anaplastic lymphoma kinase)] [136].

4.4   Lipidomics Profiling

Lipidomics is a relatively new area of research, and is now increasingly utilized due to development of novel technologies such as the time-of-flight secondary-ion mass spectrometry (TOF-SIMS) [137]. Detection of key enzymes involved in lipid metabolism, such as stearoyl-CoA desaturase 1, may also provide a signature for monitoring lipid levels, even in single cells [138].

4.5   Functional and Metabolic Heterogeneity

Generally, the EMT spectrum of CTCs demonstrates both intrapatient and interpatient heterogeneity. Researchers have also showed that not all phenotypes within the EMT spectrum may be present; with some being fully epithelial-like or mesenchymal-like [139]. More recently, it has been hypothesized that single-cell metabolomics [140] can be a unique factor for the identification of cancer cells from blood cells. These studies may be aided by the novel integrated systems, such as the nanostructure-initiator mass spectrometry (NIMS), which will serve to reveal cancer cells that may have a higher metastatic potential [141]. However, functional and metabolic studies of CTCs are highly limited by the method of CTC enrichment, which is often stressful to the primary cancer cells and compromise cellular viability.

4.5.1   Heterogeneity in Cultured CTCs

The functional properties of CTCs can be investigated with viable CTCs. However, most CTC enrichment techniques are laborious and require harsh procedures which compromise CTC viability. Analysis of the spatial-temporal characteristics of CTCs may be possible by the establishment of short-term CTC cultures with in vitro tumorsphere assays [142], structured microwell assays [63], or long-term CTC cell lines spontaneously immortalized after >6 months in culture [72, 143]. Secretion capabilities of CTCs from various cancer types can also be investigated with a membrane-based assay that provides quantification of proteins [64]. The proliferative capabilities of CTCs vary depending on marker expression [142], as well as response to therapeutic treatment [159]. More specifically, upar+/int $\beta1-$CTC subsets are shown to expand better than other combinational subsets of CTCs, and longer treatment duration correlates with lower proliferative potential. Upar−/int $\beta1-$CTC subsets also appeared to be more mesenchymal and displayed delayed clustering.

CTC may also demonstrate varied capabilities for adhesion, albeit most studies report low adhesive capabilities of CTCs. These low adhesive properties may reflect their heightened potential for extravasation and migration. Interestingly, it has been described that low adhesive CTCs demonstrate high plasticity and may eventually adhere to form spheroids under suitable 3D gel conditions [142]. Understandably, the more mesenchymal phenotypes also demonstrate higher motility and invasiveness. Analysis of these factors and other functional phenotypes, such as the formation of invadopodia [142], may reveal valuable information of the metastatic cascade occurring in vivo.

4.5.2 Cancer Stem Cells

Technological advances have enabled isolation of rare cancer subtypes with unique properties. Cancer stem cells (CSCs) are cells present in the tumor that demonstrates heightened tumorigenic potential. They are found to demonstrate distinct protein signatures, for example, breast CSCs are recognized as CD44+/CD24– [144] or aldehyde dehydrogenase 1+ (ALDH1+) cells [12, 145]. Recently, other pluripotency factors, such as POUF51 (OCT4), have been associated with the CSC subtype [146], supporting their potential role in metastasis. CSCs are often speculated to be associated with worsened patient prognosis [147], as they are found with anti-cancer drug resistant or tolerant traits [148]. Despite the distinctive characteristics of CSCs, the clinical relevance of this rare sub-population is still unclear, and further functional analysis may help to resolve this question.

5   Discussions and Conclusion

Compared to conventional macro scale devices, microfluidics technologies have provided several advantages in the field of CTC isolation such as higher throughput, greater sensitivity, portability, and ease of operation [149]. Additionally, this technique enables manipulation of fluid and particle motion at a micron-scale that is critical for CTC enrichment considering their rare occurrence in the blood. The antibody based isolation techniques provides some inherent benefits including higher specificity, lesser leukocyte contamination and enriching viable CTCs due to minimum sample handling procedure. However, these devices suffer from low throughput (1–3 ml/h) and are dependent on the expression of specific antigen markers. Due to the occurrence of EMT, some subpopulations of CTCs might not express the epithelial markers such as EpCAM and this might lead to the loss in capture efficiency [150, 151]. Label-free approaches can overcome these drawbacks of antibody-dependent methods by isolating CTCs based on their physical properties including size, deformability and dielectric properties in an unbiased manner independent of EpCAM expression. However, these techniques are limited by the heterogeneity of the cancer cells in terms of their size (CTC size varies from 6 to 30 μm) and thereby resulting in contamination from other blood cells and decreasing the isolation purity [152].

Overall, CTC isolation devices have made rapid progress over the last decade; however, till date there are few FDA approved methods (the CellSearch system and cobas EGFR Mutation Test) [153] for clinical diagnosis. Therefore, development of universal optimal protocol for examining the performances of these different devices is essential. Recent advancement of microfluidics technology has paved the way for solving some of the initial problems associated with conventional macroscale systems such as lower throughput, purity and sensitivity. The development of hybrid systems such as CTC-iChip that uses the advantages of both antibody-dependent and label-free approaches might overcome the limitations associated with both these systems individually. Additionally, negative selection devices that rely on the depletion of leukocytes may be an alternative unbiased approach for CTC enumeration. In future, we envision the development of an integrated, fully automated CTC enrichment platform that can isolate the CTCs from a simple blood test, characterize their biochemical and biophysical properties and identify the potential targets for chemotherapeutic administration.

Cancer manifests as a heterogeneous disease in several different ways [154], and detailed profiling of this manifestation is essential to develop personalized drug therapeutic strategies [155]. Biopsies of tumors are generally undesirable due to the invasive nature and possibility of dissociation of cancer cells during the surgical process. Hence CTCs represent an alternative source of cancer cells obtained via blood withdrawal, so termed as liquid biopsy [155]. The CTCs may also provide a better profile for the tumors, as they are shed from a range of sites as compared to a single biopsied region.

Several questions remain which impede the clinical utility of CTCs. The relevance of CTCs in influencing therapeutic strategies is in question since it is not known how CTCs persist within the circulation and contribute to metastasis. CTC lifespan has also not been conclusively defined, and it is speculated that this may vary from a few hours to years [156, 157]. The persistence of CTCs in blood fuels the conjecture that these rare cells may play a role in tumor relapse. Overall, the clinical relevance of CTCs will be determined by their resemblance to the original tumor phenotype, their transition in blood and their functional dynamics with time. CTCs and associated markers (e.g. microRNAs) could help to rectify the incomplete tumor profile. The characterization of CTC components may shed light for a single pathway [158] or on the patient conditions at a point of time during treatment, but monitoring of a patient's condition will require serial sampling or culturing of CTCs which could reveal dynamics of an individual's cancer progression.

Acknowledgments B.L.K. acknowledges support from the National Research Foundation (NRF), Prime Minister's Office, Singapore, under CREATE, Singapore-MIT Alliance for Research and Technology (SMART) BioSystems and Micromechanics (BioSyM) IRG and MBI. P.K.C. acknowledges the support from the Mechanobiology Institute (MBI) for the Graduate Scholarship. We thank Mr. Wong Chun Xi (MBInfo) for helping with the illustrations.

References

1. Allen JE, El-Deiry WS (2010) Circulating tumor cells and colorectal cancer. Curr Colorectal Cancer Rep 6(4):212–220
2. Majid EW, Lim CT (2013) Microfluidic platforms for human disease cell mechanics studies. In: Buehler MJ, Ballarini R (eds) Materiomics: multiscale mechanics of biological materials and structures. Springer, New York, pp 107–119
3. Chaudhuri PK et al (2016) Microfluidics for research and applications in oncology. Analyst 141(2):504–524
4. Low WS, Wan Abu Bakar WA (2015) Benchtop technologies for circulating tumor cells separation based on biophysical properties. BioMed Res Int 2015:239362
5. Alix-Panabières C, Pantel K (2014) Technologies for detection of circulating tumor cells: facts and vision. Lab Chip 14(1):57–62
6. Zabaglo L et al (2003) Cell filtration-laser scanning cytometry for the characterisation of circulating breast cancer cells. Cytometry A 55(2):102–108
7. Allard WJ et al (2004) Tumor cells circulate in the peripheral blood of all major carcinomas but not in healthy subjects or patients with nonmalignant diseases. Clin Cancer Res 10(20):6897–6904
8. Zheng S et al (2011) 3D microfilter device for viable circulating tumor cell (CTC) enrichment from blood. Biomed Microdevices 13(1):203–213
9. Zhou MD et al (2014) Separable bilayer microfiltration device for viable label-free enrichment of circulating tumour cells. Sci Rep 4:7392
10. Adams DL et al (2014) The systematic study of circulating tumor cell isolation using lithographic microfilters. RSC Adv 4(9):4334–4342
11. Chung J et al (2012) Microfluidic cell sorter (μFCS) for on-chip capture and analysis of single cells. Adv Healthcare Mater 1(4):432–436
12. Khoo BL et al (2014) Clinical validation of an ultra high-throughput spiral microfluidics for the detection and enrichment of viable circulating tumor cells. PLoS One 9(7), e99409
13. Hou S et al (2013) Capture and stimulated release of circulating tumor cells on polymer-grafted silicon nanostructures. Adv Mater 25(11):1547–1551
14. Saucedo-Zeni N et al (2012) A novel method for the in vivo isolation of circulating tumor cells from peripheral blood of cancer patients using a functionalized and structured medical wire. Int J Oncol 41(4):1241–1250
15. Tan SJ et al (2009) Microdevice for the isolation and enumeration of cancer cells from blood. Biomed Microdevices 11(4):883–892
16. Tan SJ et al (2010) Versatile label free biochip for the detection of circulating tumor cells from peripheral blood in cancer patients. Biosens Bioelectron 26(4):1701–1705
17. Desitter I et al (2011) A new device for rapid isolation by size and characterization of rare circulating tumor cells. Anticancer Res 31(2):427–441
18. Vona G et al (2000) Isolation by size of epithelial tumor cells: a new method for the immunomorphological and molecular characterization of circulating tumor cells. Am J Pathol 156(1):57–63
19. Kuo JS et al (2010) Deformability considerations in filtration of biological cells. Lab Chip 10(7):837–842
20. Alunni-Fabbroni M, Sandri MT (2010) Circulating tumour cells in clinical practice: methods of detection and possible characterization. Methods 50(4):289–297
21. Shim S et al (2013) Antibody-independent isolation of circulating tumor cells by continuous-flow dielectrophoresis. Biomicrofluidics 7(1):011807
22. Huang C-T et al (2012) Selectively concentrating cervical carcinoma cells from red blood cells utilizing dielectrophoresis with circular ITO electrodes in stepping electric fields. J Med Biol Eng 33(1):51–58
23. Gupta V et al (2012) ApoStream™, a new dielectrophoretic device for antibody independent isolation and recovery of viable cancer cells from blood. Biomicrofluidics 6(2):024133

24. Loutherback K et al (2012) Deterministic separation of cancer cells from blood at 10 mL/min. AIP Adv 2(4):042107
25. Sollier E et al (2014) Size-selective collection of circulating tumor cells using Vortex technology. Lab Chip 14(1):63–77
26. Hou HW et al (2013) Isolation and retrieval of circulating tumor cells using centrifugal forces. Sci Rep 3
27. Warkiani ME et al (2014) Slanted spiral microfluidics for the ultra-fast, label-free isolation of circulating tumor cells. Lab Chip 14(1):128–137
28. Lee MG et al (2013) Label-free cancer cell separation from human whole blood using inertial microfluidics at low shear stress. Anal Chem 85(13):6213–6218
29. Zborowski M, Chalmers JJ (2011) Rare cell separation and analysis by magnetic sorting. Anal Chem 83(21):8050–8056
30. Fehm T et al (2009) Detection and characterization of circulating tumor cells in blood of primary breast cancer patients by RT-PCR and comparison to status of bone marrow disseminated cells. Breast Cancer Res 11(4):R59
31. Punnoose EA et al (2010) Molecular biomarker analyses using circulating tumor cells. PLoS One 5(9), e12517
32. Hoshino K et al (2011) Microchip-based immunomagnetic detection of circulating tumor cells. Lab Chip 11(20):3449–3457
33. Pamme N (2012) On-chip bioanalysis with magnetic particles. Curr Opin Chem Biol 16(3):436–443
34. Kang JH et al (2012) A combined micromagnetic-microfluidic device for rapid capture and culture of rare circulating tumor cells. Lab Chip 12(12):2175–2181
35. Wang S, Owens GE, Tseng HR (2011) Nano "fly paper" technology for the capture of circulating tumor cells. Methods Mol Biol 726:141–150
36. Lu J et al (2010) Isolation of circulating epithelial and tumor progenitor cells with an invasive phenotype from breast cancer patients. Int J Cancer 126(3):669–683
37. Smith JP et al (2012) Microfluidic transport in microdevices for rare cell capture. Electrophoresis 33(21):3133–3142
38. Nagrath S et al (2007) Isolation of rare circulating tumour cells in cancer patients by microchip technology. Nature 450(7173):1235–1239
39. Stott SL et al (2010) Isolation of circulating tumor cells using a microvortex-generating herringbone-chip. Proc Natl Acad Sci 107(43):18392–18397
40. Sheng W et al (2014) Capture, release and culture of circulating tumor cells from pancreatic cancer patients using an enhanced mixing chip. Lab Chip 14(1):89–98
41. Yoon HJ et al (2013) Sensitive capture of circulating tumour cells by functionalized graphene oxide nanosheets. Nat Nanotechnol 8(10):735–741
42. Ozkumur E et al (2013) Inertial focusing for tumor antigen-dependent and -independent sorting of rare circulating tumor cells. Sci Transl Med 5(179):179ra47
43. Liu Z et al (2013) High throughput capture of circulating tumor cells using an integrated microfluidic system. Biosens Bioelectron 47:113–119
44. Seal S (1959) Silicone flotation: a simple quantitative method for the isolation of free-floating cancer cells from the blood. Cancer 12(3):590–595
45. Gertler R et al (2003) Detection of circulating tumor cells in blood using an optimized density gradient centrifugation. In: Allgayer H, Heiss M (eds) Molecular staging of cancer. Springer, Berlin, pp 149–155
46. Königsberg R et al (2011) Detection of EpCAM positive and negative circulating tumor cells in metastatic breast cancer patients. Acta Oncol 50(5):700–710
47. Naume B et al (2004) Detection of isolated tumor cells in peripheral blood and in BM: evaluation of a new enrichment method. Cytotherapy 6(3):244–252
48. Seal S (1964) A sieve for the isolation of cancer cells and other large cells from the blood. Cancer 17(5):637–642

49. Riethdorf S et al (2007) Detection of circulating tumor cells in peripheral blood of patients with metastatic breast cancer: a validation study of the Cell Search system. Clin Cancer Res 13(3):920–928
50. Diamandis EP (2002) Tumor markers: physiology, pathobiology, technology, and clinical applications. American Association for Clinical Chemistry, Washington
51. Cristofanilli M et al (2004) Circulating tumor cells, disease progression, and survival in metastatic breast cancer. N Engl J Med 351(8):781–791
52. Cristofanilli M et al (2005) Circulating tumor cells: a novel prognostic factor for newly diagnosed metastatic breast cancer. J Clin Oncol 23(7):1420–1430
53. Giordano A et al (2013) Establishment and validation of circulating tumor cell-based prognostic nomograms in first-line metastatic breast cancer patients. Clin Cancer Res 19(6):1596–1602
54. Talasaz AH et al (2009) Isolating highly enriched populations of circulating epithelial cells and other rare cells from blood using a magnetic sweeper device. Proc Natl Acad Sci 106(10):3970–3975
55. Cruz I et al (2005) Evaluation of multiparameter flow cytometry for the detection of breast cancer tumor cells in blood samples. Am J Clin Pathol 123(1):66–74
56. Yu M et al (2011) Circulating tumor cells: approaches to isolation and characterization. J Cell Biol 192(3):373–382
57. Lee HJ et al (2013) Efficient isolation and accurate in situ analysis of circulating tumor cells using detachable beads and a high-pore-density filter. Angew Chem Int Ed 52(32):8337–8340
58. McCarthy N (2014) The cancer kaleidoscope. Nat Rev Cancer 14:151–152
59. Chapman PB et al (2011) Improved survival with vemurafenib in melanoma with BRAF V600E mutation. N Engl J Med 364(26):2507–2516
60. Kwak EL et al (2010) Anaplastic lymphoma kinase inhibition in non-small-cell lung cancer. N Engl J Med 363(18):1693–1703
61. Singh AK et al (2015) Tumor heterogeneity and cancer stem cell paradigm: updates in concept, controversies and clinical relevance. Int J Cancer 136(9):1991–2000
62. Marrinucci D et al (2010) Cytomorphology of circulating colorectal tumor cells: a small case series. J Oncol 2010:861341. doi:10.1155/2010/861341
63. Khoo BL et al (2016c) Liquid biopsy and therapeutic response: circulating tumor cell cultures for evaluation of anticancer treatment. Sci Adv 2, e1600274
64. Alix-Panabieres C et al (2009) Full-length cytokeratin-19 is released by human tumor cells: a potential role in metastatic progression of breast cancer. Breast Cancer Res 11(3):R39
65. Weichselbaum RR, Hellman S (2011) Oligometastases revisited. Nat Rev Clin Oncol 8(6):378–382
66. Soslow RA et al (2012) Morphologic patterns associated with BRCA1 and BRCA2 genotype in ovarian carcinoma. Mod Pathol 25(4):625–636
67. Chen S et al (2012) Recent advances in morphological cell image analysis. Comput Math Methods Med 2012:101536
68. Gazdar AF et al (1985) Characterization of variant subclasses of cell lines derived from small cell lung cancer having distinctive biochemical, morphological, and growth properties. Cancer Res 45(6):2924–2930
69. van de Stolpe A et al (2011) Circulating tumor cell isolation and diagnostics: toward routine clinical use. Cancer Res 71(18):5955–5960
70. Leversha MA et al (2009) Fluorescence in situ hybridization analysis of circulating tumor cells in metastatic prostate cancer. Clin Cancer Res 15(6):2091–2097
71. Min JW et al (2015) Identification of distinct tumor subpopulations in lung adenocarcinoma via single-cell RNA-seq. PLoS One 10(8), e0135817
72. Zhang L et al (2013) The identification and characterization of breast cancer CTCs competent for brain metastasis. Sci Transl Med 5(180):180ra48

73. Pantel K, Alix-Panabieres C (2013) Real-time liquid biopsy in cancer patients: fact or fiction? Cancer Res 73(21):6384–6388
74. Thiery JP (2002) Epithelial-mesenchymal transitions in tumour progression. Nat Rev Cancer 2(6):442–454
75. Ting DT et al (2014) Single-cell RNA sequencing identifies extracellular matrix gene expression by pancreatic circulating tumor cells. Cell Rep 8(6):1905–1918
76. Khoo BL et al (2016) Genesis of circulating tumor cells through epithelial–mesenchymal transition as a mechanism for distant dissemination. In: Circulating tumor cells. Springer, New York, pp 139–182
77. Marrinucci D et al (2007) Case study of the morphologic variation of circulating tumor cells. Hum Pathol 38(3):514–519
78. Goda K et al (2012) High-throughput single-microparticle imaging flow analyzer. Proc Natl Acad Sci U S A 109(29):11630–11635
79. Goda K, Tsia KK, Jalali B (2009) Serial time-encoded amplified imaging for real-time observation of fast dynamic phenomena. Nature 458(7242):1145–1149
80. Navin N et al (2011) Tumour evolution inferred by single-cell sequencing. Nature 472:90–96
81. Bissell MJ, Hines WC (2011) Why don't we get more cancer? A proposed role of the microenvironment in restraining cancer progression. Nat Med 17(3):320–329
82. Michor F, Weaver VM (2014) Understanding tissue context influences on intratumour heterogeneity. Nat Cell Biol 16(4):301–302
83. Network CGA (2012) Comprehensive molecular characterization of human colon and rectal cancer. Nature 487(7407):330–337
84. Brown JM, Attardi LD (2005) The role of apoptosis in cancer development and treatment response. Nat Rev Cancer 5(3):231–237
85. Nagy P et al (1999) Activation-dependent clustering of the erbB2 receptor tyrosine kinase detected by scanning near-field optical microscopy. J Cell Sci 112(Pt 11):1733–1741
86. Tan TZ et al (2014) Epithelial-mesenchymal transition spectrum quantification and its efficacy in deciphering survival and drug responses of cancer patients. EMBO Mol Med 6(10):1279–1293
87. Pantel K, Brakenhoff RH (2004) Dissecting the metastatic cascade. Nat Rev Cancer 4(6):448–456
88. Basik M et al (2013) Biopsies: next-generation biospecimens for tailoring therapy. Nat Rev Clin Oncol 10:437–450
89. Mimeault M, Batra SK (2014) Molecular biomarkers of cancer stem/progenitor cells associated with progression, metastases, and treatment resistance of aggressive cancers. Cancer Epidemiol Biomarkers Prev 23(2):234–254
90. Borgen E et al (1999) Standardization of the immunocytochemical detection of cancer cells in BM and blood: I. Establishment of objective criteria for the evaluation of immunostained cells. Cytotherapy 1(5):377–388
91. Gollapalli K et al (2012) Investigation of serum proteome alterations in human glioblastoma multiforme. Proteomics 12(14):2378–2390
92. Francis G, Stein S (2015) Circulating cell-free tumour DNA in the management of cancer. Int J Mol Sci 16(6):14122–14142
93. Diaz LA Jr et al (2012) The molecular evolution of acquired resistance to targeted EGFR blockade in colorectal cancers. Nature 486(7404):537–540
94. Lebofsky R et al (2015) Circulating tumor DNA as a non-invasive substitute to metastasis biopsy for tumor genotyping and personalized medicine in a prospective trial across all tumor types. Mol Oncol 9(4):783–790
95. Sonnenberg A et al (2013) Dielectrophoretic isolation and detection of cfc-DNA nanoparticulate biomarkers and virus from blood. Electrophoresis 34(7):1076–1084
96. McCanna JP, Sonnenberg A, Heller MJ (2014) Low level epifluorescent detection of nanoparticles and DNA on dielectrophoretic microarrays. J Biophotonics 7(11–12):863–873

97. Bettegowda C et al (2014) Detection of circulating tumor DNA in early-and late-stage human malignancies. Sci Transl Med 6(224):224ra24
98. Diaz LA Jr et al (2013) Insights into therapeutic resistance from whole-genome analyses of circulating tumor DNA. Oncotarget 4(10):1856
99. Chan M et al (2013) Identification of circulating microRNA signatures for breast cancer detection. Clin Cancer Res 19(16):4477–4487
100. Chen X et al (2008) Characterization of microRNAs in serum: a novel class of biomarkers for diagnosis of cancer and other diseases. Cell Res 18(10):997–1006
101. Dong L et al (2014) miRNA microarray reveals specific expression in the peripheral blood of glioblastoma patients. Int J Oncol 45(2):746–756
102. Noerholm M et al (2012) RNA expression patterns in serum microvesicles from patients with glioblastoma multiforme and controls. BMC Cancer 12:22
103. Manterola L et al (2014) A small noncoding RNA signature found in exosomes of GBM patient serum as a diagnostic tool. Neuro Oncol 16(4):520–527
104. Peinado H, Lavotshkin S, Lyden D (2011) The secreted factors responsible for pre-metastatic niche formation: old sayings and new thoughts. Semin Cancer Biol 21(2):139–146
105. Costa-Silva B et al (2015) Pancreatic cancer exosomes initiate pre-metastatic niche formation in the liver. Nat Cell Biol 17(6):816–826
106. Zhao L et al (2015) The role of exosomes and "exosomal shuttle microRNA" in tumorigenesis and drug resistance. Cancer Lett 356(2):339–346
107. Chen C et al (2010) Microfluidic isolation and transcriptome analysis of serum microvesicles. Lab Chip 10(4):505–511
108. Kanwar SS et al (2014) Microfluidic device (ExoChip) for on-chip isolation, quantification and characterization of circulating exosomes. Lab Chip 14(11):1891–1900
109. Davies RT et al (2012) Microfluidic filtration system to isolate extracellular vesicles from blood. Lab Chip 12(24):5202–5210
110. Im H et al (2014) Label-free detection and molecular profiling of exosomes with a nano-plasmonic sensor. Nat Biotechnol 32(5):490–495
111. Popescu ID et al (2014) Potential serum biomarkers for glioblastoma diagnostic assessed by proteomic approaches. Proc Natl Acad Sci U S A 12(1):47
112. Skog J et al (2008) Glioblastoma microvesicles transport RNA and proteins that promote tumour growth and provide diagnostic biomarkers. Nat Cell Biol 10(12):1470–1476
113. Zhang W et al (2012) miR-181d: a predictive glioblastoma biomarker that downregulates MGMT expression. Neuro Oncol 14(6):712–719
114. Sozzi G et al (2014) Clinical utility of a plasma-based miRNA signature classifier within computed tomography lung cancer screening: a correlative MILD trial study. J Clin Oncol 32(8):768–773
115. Belting M, Wittrup A (2008) Nanotubes, exosomes, and nucleic acid-binding peptides provide novel mechanisms of intercellular communication in eukaryotic cells: implications in health and disease. J Cell Biol 183(7):1187–1191
116. Minciacchi VR, Freeman MR, Di Vizio D (2015) Extracellular vesicles in cancer: exosomes, microvesicles and the emerging role of large oncosomes. Semin Cell Dev Biol 40:41–51
117. Sun J et al (2010) A microfluidic platform for systems pathology: multiparameter single-cell signaling measurements of clinical brain tumor specimens. Cancer Res 70(15):6128–6138
118. Amir el-AD et al (2013) viSNE enables visualization of high dimensional single-cell data and reveals phenotypic heterogeneity of leukemia. Nat Biotechnol 31(6):545–552
119. Vivanco I, Sawyers CL (2002) The phosphatidylinositol 3-Kinase AKT pathway in human cancer. Nat Rev Cancer 2(7):489–501
120. Khoo BL et al (2016b) Single-cell profiling approaches to probing tumor heterogeneity. Int J Cancer 139(2):243–255
121. Dalerba P et al (2011) Single-cell dissection of transcriptional heterogeneity in human colon tumors. Nat Biotechnol 29(12):1120–1127

122. Jerome Marson V et al (2004) Expression of TTF-1 and cytokeratins in primary and secondary epithelial lung tumours: correlation with histological type and grade. Histopathology 45(2):125–134
123. Xu B et al (2010) Expression of thyroid transcription factor-1 in colorectal carcinoma. Appl Immunohistochem Mol Morphol 18(3):244–249
124. Ordonez NG (2012) Value of thyroid transcription factor-1 immunostaining in tumor diagnosis: a review and update. Appl Immunohistochem Mol Morphol 20(5):429–444
125. Lee JY et al (2015) Tumor evolution and intratumor heterogeneity of an epithelial ovarian cancer investigated using next-generation sequencing. BMC Cancer 15:85
126. Sottoriva A et al (2013) Intratumor heterogeneity in human glioblastoma reflects cancer evolutionary dynamics. Proc Natl Acad Sci U S A 110(10):4009–4014
127. Hoadley KA et al (2014) Multiplatform analysis of 12 cancer types reveals molecular classification within and across tissues of origin. Cell 158(4):929–944
128. Punnoose EA et al (2012) Evaluation of circulating tumor cells and circulating tumor DNA in non-small cell lung cancer: association with clinical endpoints in a phase II clinical trial of pertuzumab and erlotinib. Clin Cancer Res 18(8):2391–2401
129. Schiro PG et al (2012) Sensitive and high-throughput isolation of rare cells from peripheral blood with ensemble-decision aliquot ranking. Angew Chem Int Ed Engl 51(19):4618–4622
130. Lohr JG et al (2014) Whole-exome sequencing of circulating tumor cells provides a window into metastatic prostate cancer. Nat Biotechnol 32(5):479–484
131. Lacroix M (2007) Persistent use of "false" cell lines. Int J Cancer 122(1):1–4
132. Cummings EB (2003) Streaming dielectrophoresis for continuous-flow microfluidic devices. IEEE Eng Med Biol Mag 22(6):75–84
133. Baldus SE et al (2010) Prevalence and heterogeneity of KRAS, BRAF, and PIK3CA mutations in primary colorectal adenocarcinomas and their corresponding metastases. Clin Cancer Res 16:790
134. Kosmidou V et al (2014) Tumor heterogeneity revealed by KRAS, BRAF, and PIK3CA pyrosequencing: KRAS and PIK3CA intratumor mutation profile differences and their therapeutic implications. Hum Mutat 35(3):329–340
135. Deng G et al (2014) Single cell mutational analysis of PIK3CA in circulating tumor cells and metastases in breast cancer reveals heterogeneity, discordance, and mutation persistence in cultured disseminated tumor cells from bone marrow. BMC Cancer 14:456
136. Cooper WA et al (2013) Molecular biology of lung cancer. J Thorac Dis 5(Suppl 5):S479–S490
137. Ide Y et al (2014) Single cell lipidomics of SKBR-3 breast cancer cells by using time-of-flight secondary-ion mass spectrometry. Surf Interface Anal. doi:10.1002/sia.5523
138. Denbigh JL, Lockyer NP (2014) ToF-SIMS as tool for profiling lipids in cancer and other diseases. Mater Sci Technol. doi:10.1179/1743284714Y.0000000648(0)
139. Joosse SA, Gorges TM, Pantel K (2015) Biology, detection, and clinical implications of circulating tumor cells. EMBO Mol Med 7(1):1–11
140. Nemes P et al (2012) Single-cell metabolomics: changes in the metabolome of freshly isolated and cultured neurons. ACS Chem Neurosci 3:782
141. O'Brien PJ et al (2013) Monitoring metabolic responses to chemotherapy in single cells and tumors using nanostructure-initiator mass spectrometry (NIMS) imaging. Cancer Metab 1(1):4
142. Vishnoi M et al (2015) The isolation and characterization of CTC subsets related to breast cancer dormancy. Sci Rep 5:17533
143. Yu M et al (2014) Cancer therapy. Ex vivo culture of circulating breast tumor cells for individualized testing of drug susceptibility. Science 345(6193):216–220
144. Prince ME et al (2007) Identification of a subpopulation of cells with cancer stem cell properties in head and neck squamous cell carcinoma. Proc Natl Acad Sci U S A 104(3):973–978
145. Charafe-Jauffret E et al (2010) Aldehyde dehydrogenase 1-positive cancer stem cells mediate metastasis and poor clinical outcome in inflammatory breast cancer. Clin Cancer Res 16(1):45–55

146. Ennen M et al (2014) Single-cell gene expression signatures reveal melanoma cell heterogeneity. Oncogene. doi:10.1038/onc.2014.262

147. Tinhofer I et al (2014) Cancer stem cell characteristics of circulating tumor cells. Int J Radiat Biol 90(8):622–627

148. Seymour T, Nowak A, Kakulas F (2015) Targeting aggressive cancer stem cells in glioblastoma. Front Oncol 5:159

149. Whitesides GM (2006) The origins and the future of microfluidics. Nature 442(7101):368–373

150. Alix-Panabières C, Pantel K (2014) Challenges in circulating tumour cell research. Nat Rev Cancer 14(9):623–631

151. de Wit S et al (2015) The detection of EpCAM+ and EpCAM− circulating tumor cells. Sci Rep 5

152. Sun Y-F et al (2011) Circulating tumor cells: advances in detection methods, biological issues, and clinical relevance. J Cancer Res Clin Oncol 137(8):1151–1173

153. Brown P (2016) The Cobas(R) EGFR Mutation Test v2 assay. Future Oncol 12:451–452

154. Larsen JE, Minna JD (2011) Molecular biology of lung cancer: clinical implications. Clin Chest Med 32(4):703–740

155. Krebs MG et al (2014) Molecular analysis of circulating tumour cells—biology and biomarkers. Nat Rev Clin Oncol 11(3):129–144

156. Plaks V, Koopman CD, Werb Z (2013) Cancer. Circulating tumor cells. Science 341(6151):1186–1188

157. Meng S et al (2004) Circulating tumor cells in patients with breast cancer dormancy. Clin Cancer Res 10(24):8152–8162

158. Kros JM et al (2015) Circulating glioma biomarkers. Neuro Oncol 17(3):343–360

159. Khoo, BL et al (2016) Liquid biopsy and therapeutic response: Circulating tumor cell cultures for evaluation of anticancer treatment. Science Advances 2(e1600274).

The Cancer Secretome

Michaela Bowden

1 Introduction

The hallmarks of cancer provide a rational framework to evaluate the complexity and variability of cancer as a disease [1, 2]. Tumors in different organs can look much different in terms of pathology. Wide variability is observed even within a given tumor type frequently superseding differences observed across tumors. This stark reality has hindered the implementation of therapeutic options that have wide impact across large patient populations. Patients with advanced or metastatic disease have not seen appreciable improvements in overall survival rates, underlying the patient/heterogeneity paradigm that needs to be addressed in the context of the individual.

The advent of OMICS, in terms of the genome, transcriptome, proteome and metabolome has ushered in this new era of personalized cancer medicine [3–5]. The confluence of large scale measurements at the gene, protein and metabolite level, facilitated through the rapid advancement of genomics by Next Generation Sequencing (NGS) [6–8] and proteomics by Mass Spectrometry (MS) [9–11] technologies coupled with increasingly multifaceted and innovative sampling strategies [12–14] and the recognition of individual biological complexity [15, 16], has ushered in the era of personalized medicine.

Initially much focus has correctly been placed on genomic aberrations and individualized, actionable, therapeutic interventions [17–19]. In the last 10 years, the maturation of large-scale technologies has set the pace of biomarker discovery transitioning from clinical observation to a systematic approach [20]. DNA sequencing

M. Bowden (✉)
Dana Farber Cancer Institute, 450 Brookline Ave, Boston, MA 02215, USA
e-mail: michaela_bowden@dfci.harvard.edu

© Springer International Publishing Switzerland 2017
A.R. Aref, D. Barbie (eds.), *Ex Vivo Engineering of the Tumor Microenvironment,*
Cancer Drug Discovery and Development, DOI 10.1007/978-3-319-45397-2_6

and microarray techniques identify mutated or misregulated genes that are potentially druggable targets, proteomics may enable the identification of tumor-derived proteins that can serve as biomarkers of disease and response to therapy [21]. In particular, secreted or shed proteins measured in parallel, known as "secretomics" could be advantageous as early pharmacological or physiological biomarkers associated with cancer diagnosis and progression or therapeutic response and/or resistance.

In this chapter, we will describe the secreted protein oncologic landscape, the technology advancements that have facilitated the discovery and detection of the human cancer secretome, the advent of promising biomarkers and the struggle to develop them into translational clinical assays and their future utilization in personalized medicine.

2   Secreted Protein Biomarkers

2.1   What Are Secreted or "Shed" Proteins?

First described in 2000 Tjalsma et al. [22], the secretome is the term used to describe proteins shed by cells into the extracellular matrix. Over the next decade the definition was augmented to reflect the complexity of the classical and non-classical secretory mechanisms involving constitutive and regulated secretory organelles and acknowledging that secreted proteins can be shed from not only cells but tissues, organs and even organisms at any given time [23].

Secreted proteins play an important role in tumorigenesis through cell growth, migration, invasion, and angiogenesis. The main biological sources for cancer secretomics are cancer cell line supernatants and proximal biological fluids in contact with a tumor. Cancer cell line supernatant is an attractive source of secreted proteins. There are many standardized, stable cell lines and companion normal cell lines for benchmarking available. Supernatants are much simpler to analyze than proximal body fluid. But it is clear that an immortalized cell line secretome is an imperfect representation of an actual tumor, incapable of inferring information about its specific microenvironment and also not illustrative of the heterogeneity of a real tumor [24]. Analysis of proximal fluids can give a better idea of a human tumor secretome, but this method also has its drawbacks. Procedures for collecting proximal fluids still need to be standardized and non-malignant controls are needed. In addition, environmental and genetic differences between patients complicate analysis and interpretation. More recently utilizing primary tissues direct from consented patients, primary short-term cultures, patient-derived xenografts (PDX's) and patient-derived explants (PDE's) have been developed, which reconstitute and/ or preserve the inherent biological complexity as well as the heterogeneity of the patients disease.

2.2 FDA-Approved Secreted Protein Oncologic Biomarkers

Considered the gold standard in clinical quantitation of secreted biomarkers, immunoassay-based techniques including enzyme-linked immunosorbent assays (ELISA) have historically offered simplicity, cost-efficiency, selectivity, specificity, robustness and sensitivity. Most FDA-approved cancer secreted biomarkers are measured in serum and used clinically for the monitoring of disease progression and responses to therapy (e.g., CA125), the exception being prostate-specific antigen (PSA), which was approved for the detection of prostate cancer. The discovery of a large number of potential secreted cancer biomarkers in the research setting is in stark contrast to the number of markers that have been approved for use in clinical practice. Table 1 lists the handful of Food and Drug Administration (FDA) approved secreted protein biomarkers measured by immunoassay in current clinical use. There are numerous reasons why there are so few markers approved for

Table 1 List of FDA-approved protein tumor markers currently used in clinical practice, adapted from a table published by Füzéry et al. [25]

Biomarker	Clinical use	Cancer type	Year FDA approved	Device class	Product code
Pro2PSA	Discriminating cancer from benign disease	Prostate	2012	3	OYA
ROMA (HE4+CA-135)	Prediction of malignancy	Ovarian	2011	2	ONX
OVA1 (cancer antigen 125 (CA125), beta-2 microglobulin, transferrin, apolipoprotein A1 and transthyretin (prealbumin)	Prediction of malignancy	Ovarian	2009	2	ONX
HE4	Monitoring recurrence or progression of disease	Ovarian	2008	2	OIU
Fibrin/fibrinogen degradation product (DR-70)	Monitoring progression of disease	Colorectal	2008	2	NTY
CA 19-9	Monitoring disease status	Pancreatic	2002	2	NIG
CA-125	Monitoring disease progression, response to therapy	Ovarian	1997	2	LTK

(continued)

Table 1 (continued)

Biomarker	Clinical use	Cancer type	Year FDA approved	Device class	Product code
CA 15-3	Monitoring disease response to therapy	Breast	1997	2	MOI
CA 27.29	Monitoring disease response to therapy	Breast	1997	2	MOI
Free PSA	Discriminating cancer from benign disease	Prostate	1997	3	MTG
Thyroglobulin	Aid in monitoring	Thyroid	1997	3	MSW
Alpha-fetoprotein (AFP)	Management of cancer	Testicular	1992	3	LOK
Total PSA	Prostate cancer diagnosis and monitoring	Prostate	1986	2	LTJ, MTF
Carcino-embryonic antigen	Aid in management and prognosis	not specified	1985	2	DHX

clinical use, including a knowledge gap regarding study design, assay performance and the regulatory approval in the process of translating promising secretomic biomarkers from cancer discovery to diagnostics. OVA1 is the first and the only FDA-cleared in vitro diagnostic multivariate index assay of proteomic biomarkers. It tests the levels of five proteins: CA125, prealbumin, apolipoprotein A1, β2-microglobulin and transferrin [26]. The Risk of ovarian malignancy algorithm (ROMA) and prostate health index (phi) are two examples of multiple markers being measured in parallel to provide a greater level of accuracy in the clinical setting. Both OVA1 and ROMA improve the performance of CA125 in predicting ovarian malignancy in patients with pelvic mass, and phi improves the performance of total PSA and free PSA in detecting prostate cancer and avoiding unnecessary biopsies [26].

In a multitude of cancer research studies, there is an emerging rationale that as our understanding of the complexity of tumor biology and microenvironment increases at an accelerated rate, antiquated assays limited to detecting single markers may have narrow applicability and utility in a clinical setting in terms of relevancy to the disease biology and the diversity of a given patient population. Patterns of markers should prove more selective and potentially more useful than individual markers.

The emerging hallmarks of cancer, an updated re-assessment and refining of the six original hallmarks of cancer by Hanahan and Weinberg was published in 2011 (Fig. 1).

They have described two emerging hallmarks and added two enabling characteristics of the hallmarks, as shown in Fig. 2. The cancer secretome will be integral in enabling better evaluation, elucidation and translation of these new emerging

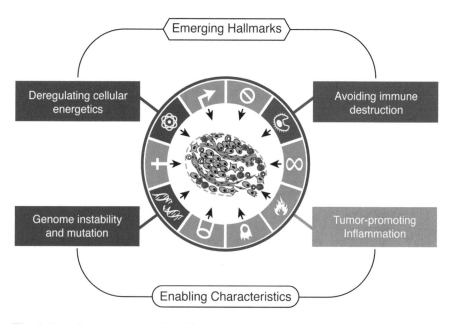

Fig. 1 Emerging hallmarks and enabling characteristics as characterized by Hanahan and Weinberg in 2011, reprinted here with permissions [2], reprinted here with permissions

hallmarks and enabling characteristics, in particular in relation to the discovery and utility of biomarkers associated with immunological evasion and pro-tumorigenic inflammatory activity.

2.3 Bead-Based Multiplexed ELISA: Targeted Profiling

The physical release of soluble cytokines and other soluble released factors from cells has now been "omed" and is called the secretome [27]. Elucidating the secretome or the cytokine network requires analysis tools that have multiplexing capability. Bead-based immunoassays read by modified flow cytometry platforms have facilitated the measurement of multiple cytokine/chemokine. A single protein will not be sufficient to fully reflect cancer complexity. Single ELISA assays in standardized 96-well plates are cumbersome and both sample exhaustive and labor-intensive. Therefore it is envisaged that a panel of secreted proteins would be more informative. Bead-based assays are dominated by xMAP® technology (Luminex Corp), which facilitates multiplexing up to 100 analytes in a single-well measurement. xMAP® uses an antibody sandwich for detection but differs from ELISA in capture substrate, substituting flat-well surface for polystyrene bead in suspension, and detection method, utilizing streptavidin-phycoerythrin fluorescent intensity

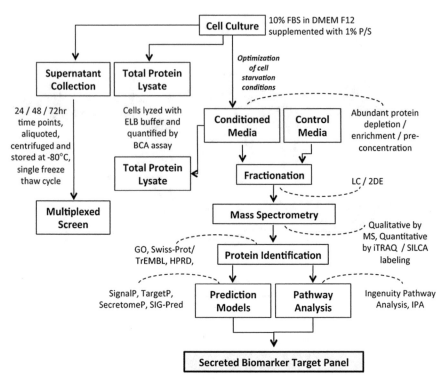

Fig. 2 Schematic of whole 'secretome' analysis workflow. Whole 'secretome analysis' comprises; conditioned media (CM) collection, CM enrichment and fractionation, proteomic separation by MS, protein identification and mapping of novel proteins to biological networks

readout. Bead-based multiplexed immunoassays provide a medium throughput, specific and reproducible analysis method that has a 3–4 logarithmic range of sensitivity compared with 1–2 logs for ELISAs [28].

Cytokines and chemokines make up a large proportion of the secretome. The immune system, including neutrophils, monocytes, macrophages, B-cells, and T-cells regulate immune responses through production of cytokines and chemokines. There are several different families of cytokine proteins including the interleukin family and chemokines, interferons, lymphokines as well as those describing functional activity such as tumor necrosis factor but generally not hormones or growth factors. Cytokines act as mediators and regulate immunological responses, hematopoietic development, and cell-to-cell communication as well as host responses to infectious agents and inflammatory stimuli. They can interact with each other in an additive, synergistic or antagonistic manner. Since cytokines work in signaling networks, it is of utmost important to be able to measure multiple cytokines in a single sample.

Over 2500 papers have been published utilizing some variation of the xMAP bead-based assays to assess cytokine, chemokine and other secreted factors in a variety of cancer models, ranging from immortalized cells lines to primary cultures to biofluids such as serum, plasma, urine and in even saliva. A few of the recent reports highlighting the utility of secretion profiling are described. Secretion of angiogenic factors, IL-6, MCP-1 and MIP-2 in ovarian spheroid cells was associated with co-culturing with adipose-derived stromal cells [29]. Th-17-related cytokines, IL-23, IL-17A, IL-17F and IL-22 were elevated in plasma from non-small cell lung carcinoma (NSCLC) patients relative to healthy donors and were associated with risk of developing NSCLC [30]. Multivariate analysis of plasma from metastatic colorectal cancer patients revealed LDH and IL-8 to be adversely prognostic in obese patients [31]. In vitro the release of TNFa, IL-6 and TGF-b by activated immune cells contributes to inflammatory breast cancer (IBC) aggressiveness [32]. Another breast study showed that plasma VEGF and MMP-9 correlate with clinical stage of breast infiltrative ductal carcinoma (IDC), tumor size and lymph node metastatic static [33]. In prostate cancer CCL-5 and PDGFRR secretion increased with increasing PIM-1 expression in co-cultures of BPH-1 epithelial cells and prostate fibroblasts, where the resultant increased myodifferentiation led to the development of cancer-associated fibroblasts in vitro [34]. Serum CCL2 was also proposed as a diagnostic biomarker of prostate cancer [35]. Urine levels of IL-8, MMP-9 and VEGF were proposed as viable diagnostic markers of bladder cancer [36] and saliva levels of IL-6 and IL-1b was markers of oral squamous cell carcinoma [37].

3   The Advent of the Proteomic Era

In 2001, the Human Proteome Organization (HUPO) initiated the Human Proteome Project (HPP) to map the entire human proteome. A cornerstone of this global effort was to adapt and implement mass spectrometry as the prime discovery platform to assess the complexity of the whole human proteome [5]. Improvements in terms of sample processing, instrumentation, data handling and informatics of MS-based proteomic approaches has resulted in increasing utility for clinical applications offering unprecedented sensitivity, specificity and throughput. Proteins perform cellular functions essential to health and/or disease. Disseminating the protein composition and disruptions in expression levels in association with a diseased state is vital to advance translational studies towards a fully personalized medicine approach.

Immunoassays measure proteins indirectly with antibodies. MS involves direct measurement of an exact peptide sequence facilitating the identification of unknown peptides with a greater degree of confidence. Immunoassays are the current gold standard in clinical detection of protein biomarkers. However the shorter lead-time, lower costs, multiplexing capabilities and flexibility in terms of configuration support MS as a powerful clinical tool.

Oncoproteomics is the study of cancer-associated proteins and their interactions using proteomic-based technologies. The routine clinical usage of proteomics to perform diagnostic and prognostic testing for determining disease status, whilst also monitoring drug toxicity and efficacy, is the ultimate goal of this field of research.

Sensitive and specific biomarkers in the detection, diagnosis, prognosis, prediction of treatment response, or monitoring of treatment are vital to clinical cancer management. In particular, early detection and intervention is typically associated with significantly improved patient outcomes. The paradigm of a single drug having therapeutic applicability to a particular cancer disease is archaic and the advent of personalized medicine suggests that single biomarkers are likely less effective than panels of biomarkers would better inform the individual's status and response to different drugs.

3.1 Cancer Secretomics: The Whole Secretome

Most secretome studies to date are performed in vitro on cultured cells, which may not directly correlate to the in vivo environment but at least immortalized cell lines cancer cell lines are very tolerant to the serum free conditions typically required to evaluate their secretome. Predominantly discovery-scale assessment of cell culture supernatant secreted proteins is carried out utilizing a mass-spectrometry approach.

Undertaking a broader-based, discovery proteomics-based approach will enhance the ability to discover clinically-relevant biomarkers [38]. Secreted proteins are excellent candidate serological tumor biomarkers and drug targets for cancer treatment [39]. Mechanistic elucidation of the corresponding signaling pathways involved could also lead to a more targeted approach to current patient treatment options in a wide variety of cancers and subtypes within a disease group. Current trends indicate that a more thorough investigation of the tumor secretome results in more sophisticated combinatorial drug approaches. Two-dimensional gel electrophoresis coupled with protein identification by mass spectrometry is the most commonly implemented approach to discovering the cancer secretome [40]. To date a standardized procedure for selection of secreted proteins as potential clinical biomarkers does not exist in the field. However the most documented approach involves focusing on differential expression of secreted proteins under two distinct conditions. Proteomic techniques are universally employed to investigate the cancer secretome. With improvements in mass spectrometry methods, comprehensive bioinformatic tool development and expansion of analytical techniques to handle clinical specimens, proteomic approaches promote the discovery of cancer secretome biomarkers [41].

3.2 Conditioned Media Sample Preparation and Purification

Incubation of cancer cells in serum-deprived media is required to eliminate abundant serum proteins that mask the lower abundance secreted proteins under investigate. However serum starvation imparts metabolic stress on the cells, resulting in reduced cell proliferation, activation of apoptotic pathways and in certain cases induction of survival mechanisms that support tumor growth [42]. Cancer cells are typically cultured in 10 % fetal bovine serum (FBS) until 70 % confluency has been reached. After which cells are washed in serum-free media or PBS and then incubated in serum-free media at 37 °C for typically 24–48 h. This conditioned media is collected, filtered and the supernatant stored at −80 °C to reduce protease activity.

Proteins are secreted by cells in vitro into conditioned media and in vivo into blood, urine, saliva etc at very low concentrations. There are also profound masking effects from serum proteins, such as albumin, extracellular proteins, fibronectin and fibulin-1 and intracellular proteins, which result in the need to purify and then concentrate the sample. Precipitation using trichloroacetic acid and ultrafiltration using molecular weight columns are most commonly employed. More recently commercially available hollow fiber culture (HFC) systems have been adapted to collect and concentrate secreted proteins [43].

3.3 Secreted Protein and Peptide Detection and Identification

Conventional and novel separation and detection techniques have been employed to interrogate the cancer secretome, where the vast majority of studies employ two-dimensional electrophoresis coupled with protein identification by mass spectrometry [44]. Differentially expressed proteins are detected Reproducibility and quantification advancements have promoted this approach. In particular, absolute quantification methodologies, such as isobaric tag for relative and label-based absolute quantitation (iTraq) and stable isotope labeling by amino acids in cell culture (SILAC) have transformed proteomics and are subject to several key reviews [45–50].

In Fig. 2, a schematic representation of a generalized workflow for whole 'secretome' analysis in cancer cells lines is presented. In parallel collecting standard supernatants and conducting secretion profiling by bead-based ELISA is hypothesized to provide a route to quickly screen for secreted proteins and to facilitate an independent methodology by which novel secreted biomarkers discovered via mass-spectrometry can be validated and translated into clinically-relevant assays that can be performed in a clinical setting that does not require specialized, expensive technology platforms and expertise to perform [51].

3.4 Cancer Cell Secretome

To date secretomic analysis of conditioned media from cancer cell lines has identified potential new biomarkers in many cancer types, including lung cancer [52–56], liver cancer [57], pancreatic cancer [58], melanoma [59], gastric cancer [60], colorectal cancer [61, 62], bladder cancer [63] and breast cancer [64–67] and identified key pathways associated with the cancer associated secretion. A single study by

Wu et al. [51] identified candidate serological biomarkers for cancer from the sec-
retomes of a large number of cancer cell lines, including oral cancer (OEC-M1 and
SCC-4), breast cancer (MCF-7 and MDA-MB-435S), bladder cancer (U1 and U4),
pancreatic ductal adenocarcinoma (PANC-1 and MIA-PaCa-2), lung adenocarcinoma (CL_{1-0} and CL_{1-5}), cervical cancer (C-33A and HeLa), lymphoma (Jurkat),
Hepatocellular carcinoma (Sk-Hep-1, HepG2 and Hep-3B), colorectal cancer
(Colo205, SW480 and SW620), skin cancer (A-431) and nasopharyngeal cancer
(NPC-TW02, NPC-TW04 and NPC-BM1), whereby they identified a wide range of
cancer-type specific candidate markers, close to 100 pan-cancer marker candidates
and proteins putatively linked to cancer-relevant pathways. Another pan-cancer
study by Wu et al. evaluated 21 cancer cell lines covering 12 cancer-types by SDS-
PAGE coupled to MALDI-TOF MS [68]. 14 proteins [alpha enolase, cyclophilin A,
heat shock protein (HSP) 90 alpha, heat shock cognate 71 kDa protein, triosephos-
phate isomerase, fructose-bisphosphate aldolase A, alpha actinin 4, cyclophilin B,
GAPDH, GRP78, phosphoglycerate mutase 1, pyruvate kinase M1/M2, Mac-2
binding protein, and cystatin C] were detected in at least 10 of the 21 cancer cell
lines. In particular elevated secretion of cyclophilin A and alpha actinin 4 were
observed in the vast majority of the cancer cell secretomes representing the potential for pan-cancer secretomic biomarkers. These seminal pan-cancer studies produced valuable databases for secretomic mapping and for future baseline
comparisons with patient-based specimens.

There has been explosion of cancer-type specific secretomic profiling studies,
where a vast amount of secreted proteins have been identified and evaluated as
potential biomarkers of malignancy, prognosis, progression, recurrence and metastasis. A selection of seminal studies that advanced the field is demonstrated here.
Kawanishi et al. compared the poorly invasive bladder cancer cell line, RT112 to the
highly invasive T24 cells [54]. By shotgun proteomics, the chemokine CXCL1 was
found to affect the invasiveness of T24 cells, where higher expression of CXCL1 by
immunohistochemistry (IHC) was associated with higher pathologic stage of the
disease. CXCL1 expression was also validated in urine from high-grade bladder
cancer patients compared to low-grade tumors. Kulasingam et al. compared the conditioned media from three breast cell lines, MCF-10A (breast epithelial), BT-474
(non-invasive breast cancer) and MDA-MB468 (metastatic breast cancer) by 2D
LC-MS/MS, resulting in the identification of 30 proteins of interest of which 11
were independently confirmed by immunoassay [57]. Activated leukocyte cell
adhesion molecule (ALCAM) was the most promising target identified and subsequently validated in a breast carcinoma patient cohort against matched normal
healthy donors, which outperformed the classical biomarkers CA15-3 and
CEA. Planque et al. conducted a comprehensive secretomic assessment of conditioned media from small cell lung cancer cell lines, H23 (adenocarcinoma), H520
(squamous cell carcinoma), H460 (large cell carcinoma) and H1688 (small cell lung
cancer) by 2D LC-MS/MS. Elevated secretion of metalloproteinase domain-
containing protein 17 (ADAM-17), osteoprotegrin, pentraxin 3, follistatin and
tumor necrosis factor receptor superfamily member 1A were identified and validated in serum by immunoassay [46].

Although a smaller number of in vivo studies involving human-derived biofluids have been undertaken; a range of clinical studies have been reported in the literature in renal cancer [69], lung [70–72], colorectal cancer [73, 74] and breast cancers [75–77], where promising potential serological biomarkers have been proposed.

Converting these novel biomarkers to translational medicine requires extensive validation and development, which presents the next major barrier to adoption of this approach in a broader clinical setting. Even where translational medicine is the laboratory focus and handling of clinical samples is the norm, most scientists are ill-equipped for the prospect of transitioning a biomarker from discovery to clinical development phase, which is a current concern that needs to be addressed to fully take advantage of this approach.

4 Patient-Derived Cancer Models

Traditional cell culture supernatants lack the tumor-host microenvironment, which more closely approximate the cancer setting. More advantageous and conversely more challenging is the prospect of utilizing patient-derived tissue to disseminate the cancer secretome. The concept of utilizing models derived from patient tissues is rigorously under investigation in a multifaceted manner as an evolution towards a new pre-clinical model paradigm; to perform drug efficacy, to capture genomic aberrations and genetic instability and to develop substantive biomarker readouts, be they disease (predictive or prognostic); or drug (pharmcodynamic or efficacy-response) related, is underway.

4.1 Patient-Derived "Short-Term" Cultures and Xenografts (PDC's/PDX's)

Immortalized cancer cell lines do not conserve the heterogeneity of the original malignancy and also are not influenced by the proper microenvironment, both traits are integral to cancer development and treatment resistance. The limited nature of in vitro models has contributed significantly to the failure of many pre-clinical models to translate to the clinical setting [78]. Using patient tissue, with minimal manipulations, better replicates the tumor microenvironment and tumor heterogeneity. Patient-derived cell cultures are created when a portion of tumor tissue is minced in culture medium and disaggregated by overnight incubation in collagenase [79]. Cells are initially cultured in tumor-type specific medium containing 10 % fetal bovine serum (FBS), antibiotics and glutamax. Once stabilized, cells can be seeded and cultured in the absence of FBS and conditioned media/cell culture supernatants can be collected, centrifuged to remove debris and stored at −80 °C for secretomic profiling.

Patient-derived xenografts are created when a fresh piece of tissue from a patient's primary tumor is implanted orthotopically, subcutaneously or under the kidney capsules of an immunodeficient mouse [70]. PDX models are known to preserve the tumor architecture and surrounding stromal compartment at the histopathological level, and inter and intra-tumoral heterogeneity, including genomic aberrations found in the patient. PDX's are also a renewable source of tumor tissue that can be serially propagated in vivo, as well as support the derivation of additional short-term cell lines at each passage in a longitudinal fashion [80]. RNA, DNA and protein from xenograft tissue and/or short-term cell line, along with biofluids such as blood, plasma, serum, exosome (in vivo) and cell culture supernatants (in vitro) can be collected/extracted and utilized in an array of downstream applications from whole genome sequencing to secretomic profiling. There are many examples of sophisticated use of these models in oncology-based pre-clinical trials [81–83].

There are many benefits to utilizing PDX models, however it is worth remembering that they lack a fully functioning immune system, require systematic histopathological and molecular characterization with every passage and are labor-intensive to manage and long-term costs can be prohibitive [70]. Currently efforts to derive PDX with a fully representative immune microenvironment are ongoing. In the future, these models will inform personal trials that can address individual variation in response to a drug and/or the onset of resistance [21].

Emerging patient-derived models include ex vivo organotypic cultures [84], in vitro 3D cultures using scaffolds [85], generation of in vitro organoid models [86] and ex vivo explants in 3D microfluidic devices [87]. Since these models most closely approximate the tumor in vivo, it is hypothesized that novel discoveries in this setting would be most readily recapitulated in the patient population. However there is a still a long way to go in terms of certitude in how these models behaves.

5   Tumor Microenvironment

Secreted proteins are encoded by approximately 10 % of the human genome [35]. The cancer secretome is comprised of proteins released or shed from the surface of a cell, tissue or organism that are vital in differentiation, invasion, metastasis and angiogenesis by regulating cell-to-cell and cell-to-extracellular matrix interactions [32]. Primary tumors are composed of cancer cells, as well as a wide variety of stromal cells, which are recruited as active co-instigators and facilitators of malignancy. This heterotypic interaction or cross-talk between cancer cells and fibroblasts in the tumor microenvironment is mediated by a variety of soluble factors, including secreted cytokines, chemokines, growth factors and immunoregulatory cytokines [88].

5.1   Cancer-Associated Fibroblast Secretome

Tumor cells only comprise a subset of the entire secretome of the microenvironment. It is critical that the stromal cell population is investigated just as rigorously to identify novel biomarkers specific to the cell type and key stromal regulators of

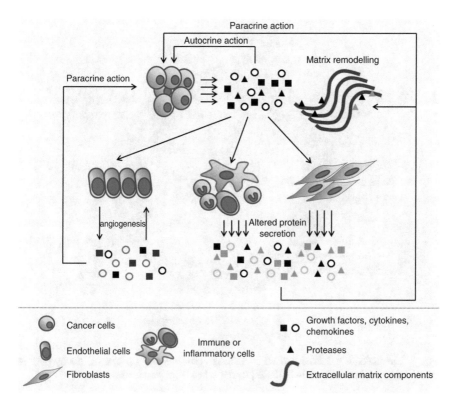

Fig. 3 Cancer secretome involving the tumor-stromal microenvironment as described by Diamandis et al. in 2010 [25], reprinted here with permissions

tumor initiation, progression and invasion [24]. By monitoring changes taking place in the tumor microenvironment via cellular and molecular profiling as malignancy progresses, the identification of cell and protein targets for cancer prevention and therapy is possible [89].

In Fig. 3, Cancer associated fibroblasts (CAF's), immune inflammatory cells such as monocytes, macrophages, neutrophils and lymphocytes and vascular endothelial cells and pericytes, as well as stromal stem and progenitor cells, comprise the entirety of the tumor microenvironment. CAF's are recruited by cancer cells to promote tumorigenesis, resulting in altered protein expression and secretion of the tumor microenvironment. CAF's provide an essential communication network via secretion of growth factors and chemokines inducing an altered extracellular matrix (ECM) [90]. They are also the most abundant cells present in tumor adjacent stroma and have distinct morphological and biological characteristics compared with normal fibroblasts. The tumor-promoting properties of CAF's can be maintained in vitro in the absence of the epithelial tumor cells. It is possible to isolate fibroblasts from primary tumor tissues and culture them in vitro to elucidate the role they play in the tumor microenvironment in a less complex biological system [91]. Reactive stroma has an increased proportion of fibroblasts present when compared with normal stroma. Invasiveness is associated with an expanding tumor stromal

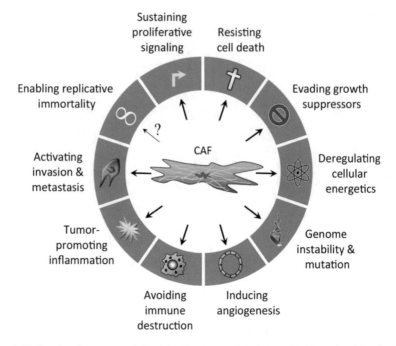

Fig. 4 Hallmarks of cancer as defined by Hanahan and Weinberg [1, 2] regulated by CAF as described by Tommelein et al. in 2015 [92] reprinted here with permissions

compartment resulting in increased deposition of ECM, known as desmoplasia. CAF's can affect cancer progression by secreting and organizing altered ECM within the tumor stroma. However the explicit transition of normal stroma into CAF's is not well understood.

Many of the original and emerging hallmarks of cancer and their enabling characteristics are interconnected and the role that CAF's play is integral to almost all of them as shown in Fig. 4. The importance of CAF's in cancer progression through multiple interactions with the cancer cells and other cell types within the tumor microenvironment suggest that secreted markers shed by CAF's could, not only further our understanding of tumor initiation and proliferation but also be targeted by novel therapeutic agents in both primary and metastatic disease.

A number of secretomic profiling studies have attempted to better understand the role CAF's play within the tumor microenvironment and what makes them different from normal fibroblasts. Chen et al. generated CAF's from fresh surgical colorectal adenocarcinoma tissue and compared them to their adjacent normal fibroblastic counterparts. Conditioned media was collected from each cell population and analyzed using SDS-PAGE, in-gel tryptic digestion and label-free LC-MS/MS. FSTL1, transgelin and decorin was found to be abundant in the fibroblastic secretome. Through silencing of transgelin and FSTL1 in the colonic fibroblast cell line CCD-18Co, enhanced colon cancer cell growth was observed in co-cultures. Independently FTSL1 was shown to have increased secretion levels in the plasma from colon cancer patients [93]. Ge et al. conducted comparative secretome analysis between CAF's and normal fibroblasts derived from differentiated nasopharyngeal squamous cell carcinoma (NPC) mucosal tissues and identified Galectin-1, a known modulator of cell-cell and cell-matrix interaction as a CAF-specific marker of influence in the context of the NPC microenvironment [94]. Bagordakis et al. expanded upon a study where a more aggressive phenotype of oral squamous cell carcinoma was directly promoted by secreted molecules from CAF's. Their study focused on examining the differences between these proliferation and invasion promoting CAF's and normal oral fibroblasts (NOF's) using label-free LC-MS/MS techniques. FNDC1, SERPINE1 and STC2 were upregulated in the CAF's and are associated with ECM organization and disassembly and collagen metabolism. Interestingly NOF's treated with TGF-β1 transformed into CAF' and expressed high levels of FNDC1, SERPINE1 and STC2 confirming their role in the CAF-derived secretome.

The secretome of myofibroblasts [61, 95] and other cell types such as macrophages [96] found in the tumor microenvironment have been studied, although there are scant examples of this in the literature.

5.2 Stem Cell Secretome

The stem cell secretome is of increasing interest to researchers, in terms of the potential use of these cells in regenerative medicine [97]. Secretomic analysis could be fundamental to understanding the underlying molecular mechanisms that drive these cells ability to self renew and differentiate. Most efforts to date have targeted characterizing growth factors, cytokine and other molecules secreted by stem cells to elucidate the immunomodulatory, anti-inflammatory and angiogenic processes [98]. A review of the stem cell secretome by Makridakis et al. highlights studies encompassing human embryonic stem cells (hESC's) [99, 100], human bone marrow derive mesenchymal stromal stem cells (hBMSC's) [101, 102], human adipose derived stem cells (hASC's) [103, 104] and cancer stem cells (CSC's) [105]. There is evidence to suggest there are glioblastoma stem cells (GSC's) capable of self-renewal that show resistance to current glioblastoma therapeutic intervention. Thriant et al. discovered hapatome derived growth factor (HDGF) was upregulated in GSC's but not in the tumor tissue itself, nor in neural stem cells (NSC's), also part of the glioblastoma tumor microenvironment. In vivo GSC's secretome induced neoangiogenesis, an effect that could be blocked by HDGF silencing by small interfering RNAs (siRNAs) [96]. Brandi et al. defined a secretomic signature of pancreatic cancer stem-like cells (CSC's) by comparing Panc1 CSC's with the parental pancreatic cell line [106]. Ceruloplasmin (CP), galectin-3 (GAL3) and MARCKS were found to be upregulated in the CSC's and were validated by immunoassay in sera from a pancreatic ductal adenocarcinoma (PDAC) patient. They propose CP as a promising marker for patients negative for CA19-9. In order to make a tangible impact, continuing advances in proteomic techniques, coupled with more sophisticated experimental design through the establishment of valid model systems is required [89].

5.3 Metastatic Secretome

Patient survival odds decrease dramatically when cancer progresses to the formation of metastatic tumors. This multistep process involves circulating tumor cells disseminating from the primary tumor and colonizing other organs. Primary tumors secrete growth factors and chemokines that mobilize inflammatory immune cells to the target organ to form this niche. The cells that comprise the niche then secrete factors both proximally and distally attracting circulating tumor cells. Better understanding of the crosstalk between immune cells at the niche and tumor cells is vital. Bidirectional crosstalk within the microenvironment at the tumor-host interface is also relevant in the metastatic setting, where tissue remodeling and adaptation is extensive. Evaluation and identification of the secreted signaling proteins that orchestrate these biological processes is an area of increased focus in recent years.

Paulitschke et al. conducted shotgun proteome and secretome profiling by MS on normal human skin fibroblasts and melanoma-associated fibroblasts from metastatic human melanoma mouse xenograft model, M24met [38]. Short-term ex vivo primary cell cultures from the fresh tissues were developed to obtain the appropriate biospecimen for subsequent analysis. A novel secreted protein, epididymal secretory gluthathione peroxidase (GPK5) was exclusively expressed by M24met melanoma cells, as well as periostatin and stanniocalcin-1 by the melanoma-associated fibroblasts. All three secreted proteins are candidate diagnostic markers that potentially could aid early detection of metastatic melanoma.

Additional studies have been undertaken to identify extracellular protein factors that modulate the metastatic phenotype of non-small cell lung cancer (NSCLC) by quantitative secretomic analysis [107], and to evaluate the cooperation between CSC and non-CSC prostate cancer cell subpopulations in driving metastasis [108].

In 2016, close to 250,000 people are projected to be diagnosed with breast cancer and almost 41,000 will develop metastasis and die in the US [109]. Almost 70 % of metastatic breast cancer is found in the bone. Secreted proteins mediate communication and interactions between metastatic cancer cells and bone stroma, as part of the broader "seed and soil hypothesis" put forward by Paget [110]. The process by which cancer cells disseminate is highly-controlled but there is still a gap in understanding exactly what cellular and molecular processes are regulating the movement of these disseminated cancer cells and their survival within the bone [111]. Combining in vitro secretomic findings from metastatic cell lines with functional validation in in vivo models is an experimental prerequisite to evaluating this complex biological system. Blanco et al. conducted a bone metastasis secretome study by SILAC-based MS to identify and annotated candidate secreted biomarkers by comparing parental breast cell lines (MDA-MB-231 and 4T1) and their metastatic derivatives. They also included in vivo experimental validation of the novel functional importance of clinically-important markers, including cathepsin inhibitors (CST1, −2 and −4), collagen functionality proteins (PLOD2 and COL6A1) and plasminogen activators (PLAT and PLAU) that have the potential to be utilized in the detection of bone metastasis as well as druggable targets for treatment [112]. Aguado et al. combined secretomic profiling and transcriptional activity as measured via Transcriptional Activity CELL aRray (TRACER) to assess the bone homing mechanism in diseased splenocyte conditioned media (D-SCM) containing immune cell secreted factors, derived from an MDA-MB-231 metastatic breast cancer mouse model [113]. Interaction between the immune cell secretome and the active transcript factors within the metastatic cells aided identification of several key functional mediators of homing, including haptoglobin, which was validated in vitro and in vivo as a tumor cell recruitment secreted factor. These two examples highlight a more systems biology approach to discovering functionally-relevant markers for metastatic processes.

6 The Advent of Personalized Medicine

Personalized medicine encompasses genomic, proteomic, transcriptomic, metabolomic and emerging—omic profiling, melded with histopathological insights to the type, stage, and grade of the disease, to individualize therapeutic intervention and/ or response to a specific drug regimen [3]. The importance of each individual— omic approach cannot be understated. The rapid advancement of high-throughput technologies, such as NGS and MS facilitate the generation of large-scale whole genome, exome and proteome data sets with a high resolution at increasingly affordable cost [3]. In order to fully utilize these platforms, technical acumen at the bench, as well as bioinformatic expertise are essential. These two areas are now particularly in an exponential phase of innovation, with respect to clinical specimen handling, sample preparation and increasingly smaller yields as input and dynamic pipeline tool augmentation and development. Targeted measurements and their integration into a pan-omics measurement is a critical step in elucidating the complexity of cancer biology systems [114].

Since the introduction of the first massively parallel DNA sequencing platforms in 2005 ushered in the new era of NGS, the rate of publication of—omic based studies associated with precision medicine has been on the rise. Based upon the last few years, we could be headed into an exponential phase of discovery as proteomic and metabolomic technologies mature and emerging—omic methods are adopted (Fig. 5).

NGS has become the standard technology and Buermans description as a molecular microscope that has been widely adopted across every field of biomedical research is very apt [8]. The ease of use and lower costs revolutionized genomics research bringing NGS into many small-scale laboratories. In parallel gene expression studies migrated from hybridization array platforms, where a priori knowledge of gene sequences was required to develop gene-specific probes for capture, to NGS, where novel transcripts could be read and mapped, and splicing, fusion and translocations could be identified [6, 7].

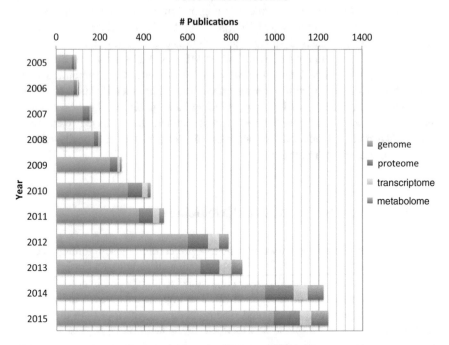

Fig. 5 Number of publications describing personalized medicine and integrated "omics", genome, proteome, transcriptome and metabolome. Bar graph showing the number of articles describing the personalized medicine field over the last decade from 2005 to 2015. NCBI Pubmed query using personalized medicine, "omics" discipline and publication year, was used to obtain data

6.1   Proteogenome

Proteomic technologies have also matured in the last decade to a level where MS delivers system-wide data on the qualitative and quantitative abundance of proteins and peptides. Proteogenomics involves the integration of genome and proteome data to facilitate more meaningful insight into the connection between physiology and genotype [10]. This field is associated with annotating newly sequenced genomes that can then be validated by MS-based proteomics data. Inclusion of RNAseq data further augments discriminating proteoforms [115, 116]. Proteogenomics faces challenges in terms of sheer scale of data generation. Developing bioinformatic tools to generate a peptide database from a given genome and then match peptides to MS/MS spectra and to merge transcriptomic and proteomic datasets to identify novel proteins and discriminate protein-coding from non-coding genes are highly desirable with the ultimate objective being correlating phenotype to genotype [107]. High profile large-scale studies are moving forwards towards integrative systems biology approaches [117, 118].

6.2 Clinically Actionable Target Identification

In 2011 the National Academy of Sciences released a framework for development of a new taxonomy of disease, a blueprint to facilitate precision medicine [12]. Putative predictive, prognostic and pharmacogenomic cancer biomarkers should support decision-making with respect to what the therapeutic options are, who would benefit from the treatment and what dose of drug would be efficacious. Countless potential cancer biomarkers have been proposed but the actual number of clinically applied predictive biomarkers is extremely low. NGS has facilitated the identification of putative targets for novel molecularly targeted therapies, such as PTEN deletion in prostate cancer and others [119]. ALK rearrangements in lung cancer and neuroblastoma [17, 120], FGFR mutation, amplification or rearrangement in many cancers including breast [121], MDM2 amplification in sarcoma [122] and MET amplification in bladder, gastric and renal cancer [123] to name a few. This list is rapidly growing as studies expand in scope and scale, incorporating many more clinical subtypes.

The human protein reference database (HPRD), mulit-omics profiling expression database (MOPED) and proteomics database (Proteomics DB) house large protein data sets, a majority of which as secretome profiles from biological fluids, which are advantageous for biomarker lead prioritization because expression levels of a target can be readily measured and monitored in responsive to therapy in a non-invasive way [24]. Only 620 of more than 22,000 proteins form the basis of mechanism-based FDA approved drugs and coalesce around a small number of protein families, including enzymes, ion channels, transporters and receptors [124], of which over 70 % are membrane-bound or secreted. Narayanan integrated chemoinformatic tools, secretomic databases and chemogenomics analysis using canSAR, a tool to mine the cancer proteome for druggability, to define 34 druggable leads, including 7 drug-like cancer bio-active lead compounds, CDC42BPB (Foretinib, a MET and VEGFR2 inhibitor), CHEK2 (CHEMBL574737, a CDK2 inhibitor), CSNK1A1 (CHEMBL2010872, a TIE-2 inhibitor), KDM4C (CHEMBL1230640, a KDM4/L3MBTL1 inhibitor), MC1R (CHEMBL373821, a melanocortin receptor inhibitor), MTPA (CHEMBL1243250, a MTAP inhibitor) and P2RY12 (CHEMBL2402259). This integration of chemogenomics and secretomics provides an immediate start point for novel therapeutic testing in primary cultures and pre-clinical models.

6.3 Integrative Systems Biology: The Revolution Will Be Personalized

In the last 5 years systems biology is transforming cancer care from symptom-based diagnosis and treatment to precision medicine. Cancer research has benefitted from whole genome and whole exome sequencing (WGS/WES). The Cancer Genome

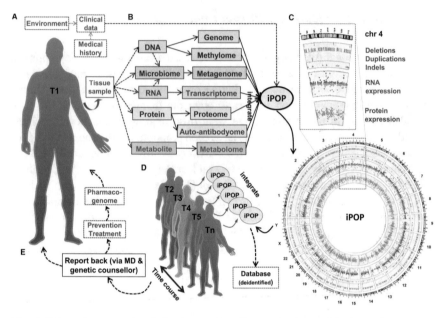

Fig. 6 Schematic representing the implementation of integrative Personal Omics Profiling (iPOP) for personalized medicine, encompassing sample collection (**a**), through omic analysis (**b**) and interpretation (**c**) to intermittent interval testing (**d**) and reporting outcome to patient (**e**), reprinted here with permissions

Atlas and the International Cancer Genome Consortium are pan-institutional collaborative initiatives to capture the genomes of all cancers. However, genomic information alone is insufficient to predict a person's health [125].

Transcriptomic, proteomic and metabolic information are a better reflection of phenotype; therefore combinatorial, longitudinal studies should elucidate an individual's physiological status. From this hypothesis the integrative Personal Omics Profie (iPOP) was first envisaged by Chen et al. [126]. iPOP is modular, allowing for additional emerging omic information to be incorporated, such as methylome, epigenome, microbiome, environome, exposome, miRNome, interactome and pharmacogenome. A schematic representation of the implementation of iPOP for personalized medicine by Li-Pook-Than is shown in Fig. 6, reprinted here with permission [127]. The first iPOP study followed a healthy individual at 20 time interval during a 14 month period through sequencing the whole genome and overlaying the exome, transcriptome, proteome, metabolome and auto-antibodyome. This analysis enabled predisposition of the individual's genetic risk and consequently tracked the early onset of type 2 diabetes in real-time [12].

Rosenblum and Peers described integrative personalized medicine as the 'the ability to look on biological systems at different "omics" levels allows us to stratify complex biological phenomena towards understanding of complex biological traits and pathologies' [5]. Ultimately monitoring patients at regular intervals and building individual omic profiles to develop molecular signatures as a real-time snapshot of the patients' physiological and pathological status. The cataloging of molecular mechanisms that confer cancer pathophysiology, serve as novel therapeutic targets, and may constitute biomarkers of early diagnosis and prediction of therapeutic response [19].

The individualized complexity that this seminal study raised revealed the very future of how disease monitoring and diagnosis should be monitored.

References

1. Hanahan D, Weinberg RA (2000) The hallmarks of cancer. Cell 100:57–70
2. Hanahan D, Weinberg RA (2011) Hallmarks of cancer: the next generation. Cell 144:646–674
3. Peer D (2014) Precision medicine—delivering the goods? Cancer Lett 352:2–3
4. Harris TJ, McCormick F (2010) The molecular pathology of cancer. Nat Rev Clin Oncol 7:251–265
5. Rosenblum D, Peer D (2014) Omics-based nanomedicine: the future of personalized oncology. Cancer Lett 352:126–136
6. Van Dijk EL, Auger H, Jaszczyszyn Y, Thermes C (2014) Ten years of next-generation sequencing technology. Trends Genet 30(9):418–426
7. Xuan J, Yu Y, Guo L, Shi L (2013) Next-generation sequencing in the clinic: promises and challenges. Cancer Lett 340:284–295
8. Buermans HPJ, den Dunnen JT (1842) Next generation sequencing technology: advances and applications. Biochim Biophys Acta 2014:1932–1941
9. Zhou L, Li Q, Wang J, Huang C, Nice EC (2015) Oncoproteomics: trials and tribulations. Proteomics Clin Appl. 2016, 10:516–31
10. Low TY, Heck AJR (2016) Reconciling proteomics with next generation sequencing. Curr Opin Chem Biol 30:14–20
11. Baker ES, Liu T, Petyuk VA, Burnum-Johnson KE, Ibrahim YM, Anderson GA, Smith RD (2012) Mass spectrometry for translational proteomics: progress and clinical implications. Genome Med 4:63
12. Simon R, Roychowdhury S et al (2013) Implementing personalized cancer genomics in clinical trials. Nat Rev Drug Discov 12:358–369
13. Gravitz L (2014) This time it's personal. Nature 509:S52–S54
14. Schork NJ (2015) Time for one-person trials. Nature 520:609–611
15. De Bono JS, Ashworth A (2010) Translating cancer research into targeted therapeutics. Nature 467:543–549
16. Haber DA, Gray NS, Baselga J (2011) The evolving war on cancer. Cell 145:19–24
17. Kwak EL, Bang YJ, Camidge DR, Shaw AT, Solomon B, Maki RG, Ou SH, Dezube BJ, Jänne PA, Costa DB, Varella-Garcia M, Kim WH, Lynch TJ, Fidias P, Stubbs H, Engelman JA, Sequist LV, Tan W, Gandhi L, Mino-Kenudson M, Wei GC, Shreeve SM, Ratain MJ, Settleman J, Christensen JG, Haber DA, Wilner K, Salgia R, Shapiro GI, Clark JW, Iafrate AJ (2010) Analplastic lymphoma kinase inhibition in non-small cell lung cancer. N Engl J Med 363(18):1693–1703
18. Chapman PB, Hauschild A, Robert C, Haanen JB, Ascierto P, Larkin J, Dummer R, Garbe C, Testori A, Maio M, Hogg D, Lorigan P, Lebbe C, Jouary T, Schadendorf D, Ribas A, O'Day SJ, Sosman JA, Kirkwood JM, Eggermont AM, Dreno B, Nolop K, Li J, Nelson B, Hou J, Lee RJ, Flaherty KT, McArthur GA (2011) Improved survival with vemurafenib in melanoma with BRAF V600E mutation. N Engl J Med 364(26):2507–2516
19. Stegh AH et al (2013) Toward personalized cancer nanomedicine—past, present, and future. Integr Biol 5:48–65

20. Pavlou PA, Diamanids EP, Blaustig IM (2013) The long journey of cancer biomarkers from the bench to the clinic. Clin Chem 59(1):1–11
21. De Palma M, Hanahan D (2012) The biology of personalized cancer medicine: facing individual complexities underlying hallmark capabilities. Mol Oncol 6(2):111–127
22. Tjalsma H, Bolhuis A, Jongbloed JD, Bron S, van Dijl JM (2000) Signal peptide-dependent protein transport in Bacillus subtilis: a genome-based survey of the secretome. Microbiol Mol Biol Rev 64:515–547
23. Agrawal GK, Jwa N-S, Lebrun M-H, Job D, Rakwal R (2010) Plant secretome: unlocking secrets of the secreted proteins. Proteomics 10(4):799–827
24. Karagiannis GS, Pavlou MP, Diamandis EP (2010) Cancer secretomics reveal pathophysiological pathways in cancer molecular oncology. Mol Oncol 4(6):496–510
25. Füzéry AK, Levin J, Chan MM, Chan DW (2013) Translation of proteomic biomarkers into FDA approved cancer diagnostics: issues and challenges. Clin Proteomics 10:13
26. Li D, Chan DW (2014) Proteomic cancer biomarkers from discovery to approval: it's worth the effort. Expert Rev Proteomics 11(2):135–136
27. Skalnikova H, Motlik J, Gadher SJ, Kovarova H (2011) Mapping of the secretome of primary isolates of mammalian cells, stem cells and derived cell lines. Proteomics 11:691–708
28. Pawlak M, Schick E, Bopp MA, Schneider MJ, Oroszlan P, Ehrat M (2002) Zeptosens' protein microarrays: a novel high performance microarray platform for low abundance protein analysis. Proteomics 2:383–393
29. Zhang Y, Nowicka A et al (2015) Stromal cells derived from visceral and obese adipose tissue promote growth of ovarian cancers. Plos One 8:U1294–U1310
30. Liao C, Yu ZB et al (2015) Association between Th17-related cytokines and risk of non-small cell lung cancer among patients with or without chronic obstructive pulmonary disease. Cancer 17:3122–3129
31. Shah MS, Fogelman DR et al (2015) Joint prognostic effect of obesity and chronic systemic inflammation in patients with metastatic colorectal cancer. Cancer 121(17):2968–2975
32. Cohen EN, Gao H et al (2015) Inflammation mediated metastasis: immune induced epithelial-to-mesenchymal transition in inflammatory breast cancer cells. PLoS One 10(7), e0132710
33. Zhang J, Yin L et al (2014) Detection of serum VEGF and MMP-9 levels by Luminex multiplexed assays in patients with breast infiltrative ductal carcinoma. Exp Ther Med 8(1):175–180
34. Zemskova MY, Song J et al (2015) Regulation of prostate stromal fibroblasts by the PIM1 protein kinase. Cell Signal 27(1):135–146
35. Tsaur I, Noack A et al (2015) CCL2 chemokine as a potential biomarker for prostate cancer: a pilot study. Cancer Res Treat 47(2):306–312
36. Rosser CJ, Dai Y (2014) Simultaneous multi-analyte urinary protein assay for bladder cancer detection. BMC Biotechnol 14:24
37. Arellano-Garcia ME, Hu S et al (2008) Multiplexed immunobead-based assay for detection of oral cancer protein biomarkers in saliva. Oral Dis 14(8):705–712
38. Paulitschke V, Kunstfeld R et al (2009) Entering a new era of rational biomarker discovery for early detection of melanoma metastases: secretome analysis of associated stroma cells. J Proteome Res 8:2501–2510
39. Madridakis M, Vlahou A (2010) Secretome proteomics for discovery of cancer biomarkers. J Proteomics 73:2291–2305
40. Dowling P, o'Driscoll L, Meleady P, Henry M, Roy S, Ballot J, Moriarty M, Crown J, Clynes M (2007) 2-D difference gel electrophoresis of the lung squamous cell carcinoma versus normal sera demonstrates consistent alterations in the levels of ten specific proteins. Electrophoresis 28:4302–4310
41. Xue H, Lu B, Lai M (2008) The cancer secretome: a reservoir of biomarkers. J Transl Med 6:51
42. Levin VA, Panchabhai SC et al (2010) Different changes in protein and phosphoprotein levels results from serum starvation. J Proteome Res 9:179–191
43. Lin Q, Tan HW et al (2013) Sieving through the cancer secretome. Biochim Biophys Acta 1834:2360–2371

44. Pavlou MP, Diamandis EP (2010) The cancer cell secretome: a good source for discovering biomarkers. J Proteomics 73:1896–1906
45. Paul D, Kumar A, Gajbhiye A, Santra MK, Srikanth R (2013) Mass spectrometry-based proteomics in molecular diagnostics: discovery of cancer biomarkers using tissue culture. Biomed Res Int 2013:783131
46. Evans C, Noirel J, Ow SY, Salim M, Pereira-Medrano AG, Couto N, Pandhal J, Smith D, Pham TK, Karunakaran E, Zou X, Biggs CA, Wright PC (2012) An insight into iTRAQ: where do we stand now? Anal Bioanal Chem 404(4):1011–1027
47. Chahrour O, Cobice D, Malone J (2015) Stable isotope labeling methods in mass spectrometry-based quantitative proteomics. J Pharm Biomed Anal 113:2–20
48. Dittmar G, Selbach M (2015) SILAC for biomarker discovery. Proteomics Clin Appl 9(3–4): 301–306
49. Chen X, Wei S, Ji Y, Guo X, Yang F (2015) Quantitative proteomics using SILAC: principles, applications, and developments. Proteomics 15(18):3175–3192
50. Stastna M, Van Eyk JE (2012) Secreted proteins as a fundamental source of biomarker discovery. Proteomics 12:722–735
51. Wu CC, Hsu CW, Chen CD, Yu CJ, Chang KP, Tai DI, Liu HP, Su WH, Chang YS, Yu JS (2010) Candidate serological biomarkers for cancer identified from the secretomes of 23 cancer cell lines and the human protein atlas. Mol Cell Proteomics 9(8):1100–1117
52. Hu R, Huffman K et al (2016) Quantitative secretomic analysis identifies extracellular protein factors that modulate the metastatic phenotype of non-small cell lung cancer. J Proteome Res 15:477–486
53. Luo X, Liu Y (2011) A high-quality secretome of A549 cells aided the discovery of C4b-binding protein ass a novel serum biomarker for non-small cell lung cancer. J Proteomics 74:528–538
54. Wang CI, Wang CW et al (2011) Importin subunit alpha-2 is identified as a potential biomarker for non-small cell lung cancer by integration of the cancer cell secretome and tissue transcriptome. Int J Cancer 128:2364–2372
55. Planque C, Kulasingam V et al (2009) Identification of five candidate lung cancer biomarkers by proteomics analysis of conditioned media of four lung cancer cell line. Mol Cell Proteomics 8(12):2746–2758
56. Wang CL, Wang CI et al (2009) Discovery of retinoblastoma-associated binding protein 46 as a novel prognostic marker for distant metastasis in non small cell lung cancer by combined analysis of cancer cell secretome and pleural effusion proteome. J Proteome Res 8:4428–4440
57. Yu Y, Pan X et al (2013) An iTRAQ based quantitative proteomic strategy to explore novel secreted proteins in metastatic hepatocellular carcinoma cell lines. Analyst 138(16):4505–4511
58. Schiarea S, Solinas G et al (2010) Secretome analysis of multiple pancreatic cancer cell lines reveals perturbations of key functional networks. J Proteome Res 9(9):4376–4392
59. Rocco M, Malorni L et al (2001) Proteomic profiling of human melanoma metastatic cell line secretomes. J Proteome Res 10:4703–4714
60. Loei H, Tan HT et al (2011) Mining the gastric cancer secretome: identification of GRN as a potential diagnostic marker for early gastric cancer. J Proteome Res 11:1759–1772
61. Karagiannis GS, Petraki C et al (2012) Proteomic signatures of the desmoplastic invasion front reveal collagen type XII as a marker of myofibroblastic differentiation during colorectal cancer metastasis. Oncotarget 3:267–285
62. Yao L, Lao W et al (2012) Identification of EFEMP2 as a serum biomarker for the early detection of colorectal cancer with lectin affinity capture assisted secretome analysis of cultured fresh tissue. J Proteome Res 11:3281–3294
63. Kawanishi H, Matsui Y et al (2008) Secreted CXCL1 is a potential mediator and marker of the tumor invasion of bladder cancer. Clin Cancer Res 14(9):2579–2587
64. Jeon YR, Kim SY et al (2013) Identification of annexin II as a novel secretory biomarker for breast cancer. Proteomics 13:3145–3156

65. Chevalier F, Depagne J et al (2013) Accumulation of cyclophilin A isoforms in conditioned media of irradiated breast cancer cells. Proteomics 12:1756–1766
66. Kulasingam V, Zheng Y et al (2009) Activated leukocyte cell adhesion molecule: a novel biomarker for breast cancer. Int J Cancer 125:9–14
67. Whelan SA, He J et al (2012) Mss Spectrometry (LC-MS/MS) identified proteomic biosignatures of breast cancer in proximal fluid. J Proteome Res 11:5034–5045
68. Wu CC, Chen HC et al (2008) Identification of collapsing response mediator protein-2 as a potential marker of colorectal carcinoma by comparative analysis of cancer cell secretomes. Proteomics 8:316–332
69. Sandim V, Pereira DA et al (2016) Proteomic analysis reveals differentially secreted proteins in the urine from patients with clear cell renal cell carcinoma. Urol Oncol Sem Orig Invest 34:5.e11–e25.
70. Wang Z, Wang C et al (1824) Differential proteome profiling of pleural effusions from lung cancer and benign inflammatory disease patients. Biochim Biophys Acta 2012:692–700
71. Li Y, Lian H et al (2015) Proteome screening of pleural effusions identifies IL1A as a diagnostic biomarker for non-small cell lung cancer. Biochem Biophys Res Commun 457(2):177–182
72. Xiao H, Zhang H et al (2012) Proteomic analysis of human saliva from lung cancer patients using two-dimensional difference gel electrophoresis and mass spectrometry. Mol Cell Proteomics 11:M111
73. Fijneman RJ, de Wit M et al (2012) Proximal fluid proteome profiling of mouse colon tumors reveals biomarkers for early diagnosis of human colorectal cancer. Clin Cancer Res 18:2613–2624
74. Ang CS, Rothacker H et al (2011) Use of multiple reaction monitoring for multiplex analysis of colorectal cancer-associated proteins in human feces. Electrophoresis 32:1926–1938
75. Gromov P, Gromova I et al (2010) Up-regulated proteins in the fluid bathing the tumor cell microenvironment as potential serological markers for early detection of cancer of the breast. Mol Oncol 4:65–89
76. Raso C, Cosentino C et al (2012) Characterization of breast cancer interstitial fluids by TnT labeling, LTQ-orbitrap velos mass spectrometry, and pathway analysis. J Proteome Res 11:3199–3210
77. Alexander H, Stegner AL et al (2004) Proteomic analysis to identify breast cancer biomarkers in nipple fluid. Clin Cancer Res 10:7500–7510
78. Choi SYC, Lin D et al (2014) Lessons from patient-derived xenografts for better in vitro modeling of human cancer. Adv Drug Deliv Rev 79–80:222–237
79. Baguley BC, Marshall ES (1999) Short-term cultures of clinical tumor material: potential contributions to oncology research. Oncol Res 11:115–124
80. Tentler JJ, Tan AC et al (2012) Patient-derived tumor xenografts for oncology drug development. Nat Rev Clin Oncol 9:338–350
81. Lee JY, Kim SY et al (2015) Patient-derived cell models as preclinical tools for genome-directed targeted therapy. Oncotarget 6(28):25619–25630
82. Girotti MR, Gremel G et al. Application of sequencing, liquid biopsies and patient-derived xenografts for personalized medicine in melanoma. Cancer Discov. 2016. doi:10.1158/2159-8290. CD-15-1336
83. Whittle JR, Lewis MT et al (2015) Patient-derived xenograft models of breast cancer and their predictive power. Breast Cancer Res 17:17
84. Naipal KA, Verkaik NS et al (2016) Tumor slice culture system to assess drug response of primary breast cancer. BMC Cancer 16:78
85. Sokol ES, Miller DH et al (2016) Growth of human breast tissues from patient cells in 3D hydrogel scaffolds. Breast Cancer Res 18:19
86. Gao D, Vela I et al (2014) Organoid cultures derived from patients with advanced prostate cancer. Cell 159:176–187
87. Zervantonakis IK, Hughes-Alford SK et al (2012) Three-dimensional microfluidic model for tumor cell intravasation and endothelial barrier function. Proc Natl Acad Sci U S A 109(34):13515–13520

88. Mishra P, Banerjee D, Ben-Baruch A (2011) Chemokines at the crossroads of tumor-fibroblast interactions that promote malignancy. J Leukoc Biol 89:31–39

89. MBeunkui F, Johann DJ et al (2009) Cancer and the tumor microenvironment: a review of an essential relationship. Cancer Chemother Pharmacol 63:571–582

90. Kalluri R, Zeisberg M (2006) Fibroblasts in cancer. Nat Rev Cancer 6(5):392–401

91. Orimo A, Gupta PB et al (2005) Stromal fibroblasts present in invasive human breast carcinomas promotes tumor growth and angiogenesis through elevated SDF-1/CXCL12 secretion. Cell 121:335–348

92. Tommelein J, Verset L, Boterberg T, Demetter P, Bracke M, De Wever O (2015) Cancer-associated fibroblasts connect metastasis-promoting communication in colorectal cancer. Front Oncol 5:63 [Open-access - Creative Commons Attribution License (CC BY)]

93. Chen S-X, Xu X-E et al (2014) Identification of colonic fibroblast secretomes reveals secretory factors regulating colon cancer cell proliferation. J Proteomics 110:155–171

94. Ge S, Mao YM et al (2012) Comparative proteomic analysis of secreted proteins from nasopharyngeal carcinoma-associated stromal fibroblasts and normal fibroblasts. Exp Ther Med 3:857–860

95. Holmberg C, Ghesquiere B et al (2013) Mapping proteolytic processing in the secretome of gastric cancer-associated myofibroblasts reveals activation of MMP_1, MMP-2 and MMP-3. J Proteome Res 12:3413–3422

96. Kobayashi R, Deavers M et al (2009) 14-3-3 zeta protein secreted by tumor-associated monocytes/macrophages from ascites of epithelial ovarian cancer patients. Cancer Immunol Immunother 58:247–258

97. Makridakis M, Roubelakis MG et al (2013) Biochim Biophys Acta 1834:2380–2384

98. Roche S, D'Ippolito G et al (2013) Comparative analysis of protein expression of three stem cell populations: models of cytokine delivery system in vivo. Int J Pharm 440:72–82

99. Sarkar P, Randall SM (2012) Targeted proteomics of the secretory pathway reveals the secretome of mouse embryonic fibroblasts and human embryonic stem cells. Mol Cell Proteomics 11:1829–1839

100. Bendall SC, Hughes JL et al (2009) An enhanced mass spectrometry approach reveals human embryonic stem cell growth factors in culture. Mol Cell Proteomics 8:421–432

101. Kim JM, Kim YH et al (2013) Comparative secretome analysis of human bone marrow-derived mesenchymal stem cells during osteogenesis. J Cell Physiol 228:216–224

102. Choi YA, Lim KM et al (2010) Secretome analysis of human BMSC's and identification of SMOC1 as an important ECM protein in osteoblast differentiation. J Proteome Res 9:2946–2956

103. Lee MJ, Kim J et al (2010) Proteomic analysis of tumor necrosis factor-alpha-induced secretome of human adipose tissue-derived mesenchymal stem cells. J Proteome Res 9:1754–1762

104. Chiellini C, Cochet I et al (2008) Characterization of human mesenchymal stem cell secretome at early steps of adipocyte and osteoblast differentiation. BMC Mol Biol 9:26

105. Thirant C, Galan-Moya EM et al (2012) Differential proteomicanalysis of human glioblastoma and neural stem cells reveals HDGF as a novel angiogenic secreted factor. Stem Cells 30:845–853

106. Brandi J, Dalla Pozza E et al (2016) Secretome protein signature of human pancreatic cancer stem-like cells. J Proteomics 136:1–12

107. Rongkuan H, Huffman KE et al (2016) Quantitative secretomic analysis identifies extracellular protein factors that modulate the metastatic phenotype of non-small cell lung cancer. J Proteome Res 15:477–486

108. Mateo F, Meca-Cortes O et al (2014) SPARC mediates metastatic cooperation between CSC and non-CSC prostate cancer cell subpopulations. Mol Cancer 13:237

109. American Cancer Society (2016) Cancer facts and figures 2016. American Cancer Society, Atlanta, GA. Also available online: Exit Disclaimer (PDF—1.67 MB). Accessed 1 Feb 2016

110. Paget S (1889) The distribution of secondary growths in cancer of the breast. Lancet 133:571–573

111. Suva LJ, Washam C et al (2011) Bone metastasis: mechanisms and therapeutic opportunities. Nat Rev Endocrinol 7(4):208–218

112. Blanco MA, LeRoy G et al (2012) Global secretome analysis identifies novel mediators of bone metastasis. Cell Res 22:1339–1355

113. Aguado BA, Wu JJ et al (2015) Secretome identification of immune cell factors mediating metastatic cell homing. Sci Rep 5:17566

114. Smith RD (2012) Mass Spectrometry in biomarker applications: from untargeted discovery to targeted verification, and implications for platform convergence and clinical application. Clin Chem 58:528–530

115. Nesvizhskii AI (2014) Proteogenomics: concepts, applications and computational strategies. Nat Methods 11:1114–1125

116. Low TY, van Heesch S et al (2013) Quantitative and qualitative proteome characteristics extracted from in-depth integrated genomics and proteomics analysis. Cell Rep 5:1469–1478

117. Weinstein JN, Collisson EA et al (2013) The cancer genome atlas pan-cancer analysis project. Nat Genet 45:1113–1120

118. Ritchie MD, Holzinger ER et al (2015) Methods of integrating data to uncover genotype-phenotype interactions. Nat Rev Genet 16L:85–97

119. Hollander MC, Blumenthal GM et al (2011) PTEN loss in the continuum of common cancers, rare syndromes and mouse models. Nat Rev Cancer 11:289–301

120. Chen Y et al (2008) Oncogenic mutations of ALK kinase in neuroblastoma. Nature 455:971–974

121. Turner N, Grose R et al (2010) Fibroblast growth factor signaling: from development to cancer. Nat Rev Cancer 10:116–129

122. Shangary S, Wnag S et al (2008) Targeting the MDM2-p53 interaction for cancer therapy. Clin Cancer Res 14:5318–5324

123. Woude G (2012) Targeting MET, in cancer: rationale and progress. Nat Rev Cancer 12:89–103

124. Narayanan R (2015) Druggable cancer secretome: neoplasm-associated traits. Cancer Genomics Proteomics 12:119–132

125. Chen R, Snyder M et al (2012) Systems biology: personalized medicine for the future? Curr Opin Pharmacol 12:623–628

126. Chen R, Mias GI et al (2012) Personal omics profiling reveals dynamic molecular and medical phenotypes. Cell 148:1293–1307

127. Li-Pook-Than J, Snyder M et al (2013) iPOP goes the world: integrated personalized omics profiling and the road toward improved health care. Chem Biol 20:660–666

The Importance of Circulating Tumor Cells and Tumor Models in Future of Cancer Therapy

Babak Behnam, Hassan Fazilaty, and Ali Roghanian

1 Introduction

Cancer-associated mortalities are mainly due to the spread of tumor cells from primary sites to secondary organs via a mysterious journey, a process called metastasis. In order to metastasize, tumor cells delaminate from the primary site and enter to the circulation (blood/lymph), through which they can travel and reach distant organs and overt secondary tumors [1]. These circulating tumor cells (CTC) have to win the battle against several different defense mechanisms of the body. The processes involved in tumor metastasis are highly complex and vastly unknown, and require understanding of the molecular mechanisms. Therefore, they have to carry out a smart well-orchestrated plastic program to progress and survive. It has been shown in several types of carcinomas that epithelial cancer cells need to go through a transition program called epithelial-mesenchymal transition (EMT), in which cuboid epithelial cells acquire mesenchymal features in order to migrate and invade

B. Behnam (✉)
NIH Undiagnosed Diseases Program, National Human Genome Research Institute (NHGRI), National Institutes of Health (NIH), Bethesda, MD 20892, USA

Department of Medical Genetics and Molecular Biology, School of Medicine, Iran University of Medical Sciences (IUMS), Tehran, Iran
e-mail: babak.behnam@nih.gov; b_behnam@yahoo.com

H. Fazilaty
Instituto de Neurociencias CSIC-UMH, San Juan de Alicante, Spain
e-mail: hfazilaty@umh.es

A. Roghanian
Antibody and Vaccine Group, Cancer Sciences Unit, Faculty of Medicine, University of Southampton, Southampton General Hospital, Southampton, UK

Koch Institute for Integrative Cancer Research, Massachusetts Institute of Technology, Cambridge, MA, USA
e-mail: a.roghanian@soton.ac.uk; aroghani@mit.edu

© Springer International Publishing Switzerland 2017
A.R. Aref, D. Barbie (eds.), *Ex Vivo Engineering of the Tumor Microenvironment*, Cancer Drug Discovery and Development, DOI 10.1007/978-3-319-45397-2_7

121

from the primary site. On the other hand, for colonization in the secondary organ, tumor cells ought to have epithelial characteristics such as high proliferation to overt metastatic tumors, which suggest a reversion of mesenchymal to epithelial state called mesenchymal-epithelial transition (MET) [2–6]. Several signaling networks and molecular mechanisms are involved in cancer metastasis and epithelial plasticity in a spatiotemporal manner [7–11]. Also, the importance of hypoxia has been well recognized in the tumor microenvironment as well as the emergence of cancer stem cells (CSC) [11, 108]. Notably overexpressed major players in hypoxia (*e.g.*, HIF-1α, BNIP3, CA-IX and GLUT1), EMT (*e.g.*, Snail, Twist, EpCam, Vimentin and E-cadherin), and CSC (*e.g.*, Nanog, OCT4 and SOX2) provide a suitable microenvironment for the CSCs and CTCs escape from immune attack in the blood stream.

One of the most promising ways to understand cancer biology is to study human derived cancer models, where primary tumors are analyzed outside their host. Among these models, cancer cell lines, PDTX and, more recently developed, primary tumor organoids are current most used models.

1.1 Immune System Suppression and Evasion by CSCs

Immune surveillance has the potential to recognize malignant cells and eliminate them in their infancy. However, cancer cells have developed strategies to evade immunity or even tolerize the immune system in order to avoid elimination by these specialized cells [12]. Hence, immune evasion by cancer cells is one of the 'hallmarks for cancer' which in recent years has attracted researchers' attention and has been the subject of intense investigation [13]. Similar to cancer cells, CSCs identified in a wide range of tumors have been shown to express/secrete a large number of immunosuppressive molecules, such as CD200 and CD47 (see below), and are poorly immunogenic, which results in their protection from the immune system [14]. Additionally, it has been suggested that CSCs may interact with the immune cells within the tumor microenvironment to "hitchhike" through the circulatory system, shielding themselves from destruction by systemic shear stress and the immune system [15]. Although still in its infancy, CSC immunology has attracted more attention in recent years and would prove to be an important and fundamental avenue to target tumor progression, dissemination and resistance in patients.

One of the most studied receptors implicated in immune evasion is CD47, which is a widely expressed cell surface protein expressed on cancer cells. Importantly, CD47 has been shown to be expressed by certain CSCs, such as primary human acute myeloid leukemia (AML) stem cells [16, 17]. Casey and colleagues recently demonstrated that CD47 expression is controlled by the MYC oncogene which binds directly to its promoter [18]. Moreover, hypoxia-inducible factor 1 (HIF-1) directly activates transcription of the CD47 gene in hypoxic breast cancer cells [19]. Increased expression of CD47 has been reported to act as a 'don't eat me' signal and, via binding to signal-regulatory protein alpha (SIRP-α), enables cancer cells to evade phagocytosis by macrophages [19, 20]. A recent study reported that, in addition to inhibiting phagocytosis, the expression of mouse CD47 receptor on human tumors can potentiate metastasis in an in vivo xenograft model [21]. In agreement with these observations, agents such as mAbs that block the CD47:SIRP-α engagement are attractive therapeutic candidates as a monotherapy or in combination with additional immunomodulating drugs for activating antitumor responses in cancer patients [22]. Similarly, targeting of CD47 by specific blocking mAbs would also be a viable strategy for eradicating CSCs [23].

Another receptor implicate in CSC immune evasion is CD200 (OX2), a highly conserved member of the immunoglobulin superfamily, which is a widely distributed cell surface protein. CD200 interacts with CD200R that is highly expressed on myeloid and some lymphoid cells, such as macrophages and activated T cells [24]. CD200 activation leads to a potent immune suppression in immune cells. For instance, CD200:CD200R engagement on macrophages suppresses cytokine production by macrophages [25]. In addition, CD200 has been shown to express on the surface of several cancer cells, such as melanoma, breast, chronic lymphocytic leukemia and ovarian cancers, and its knockdown in mice results in earlier onset of autoimmunity [26]. As such, cancer cells have been shown to downregulate immune cells activation via CD200:CD200R engagement in various experimental models [27, 28]. More importantly, CD200 has been reported to be highly upregulated in CSCs, which may function in immune evasion and suppression by these cells [29]. This makes CD200 an interesting target for targeting CSCs therapeutically [30].

Other potential CSC surface targets include CD44 and CD133 [31]. CD44 is a ubiquitously expressed transmembrane glycoprotein highly expressed by CSCs, such as breast, prostate and pancreatic CSCs. CD44 plays a major role in tumor proliferation, survival, progression and metastasis and is used for isolation of CSCs [32–35]. Hence, CD44 may be a therapeutic target for eradicating CSCs. In this regards, CD44 specific mAbs have been shown to inhibit growth of AML cells in vivo [32]. On the other hand, CD133 expression on tumor cells makes them resistant to chemo- and radio-therapy is a marker of poor prognosis [36]. CD133 mAbs have therefore been generated to successfully target CSCs in experimental models [37].

In addition to the expression of surface markers, CSCs have been shown to secrete immunosuppressive molecules. For instance, breast and glioblastoma CSCs secrete more TGF-β as compared to normal tumor cells [38, 39]. Colon CSCs are further known to secrete Interleukin 4, which promotes drug resistance [40, 41]. These cytokines are potent inducers of tolerogenic dendritic cells and M2-polarized macrophages, which are responsible for inducing immune suppression [42, 43].

In summary, as outlines above, it is clear that CSCs, via expression of numerous cell-bound and soluble factors, employ a wide range of immune evasion and/or suppressive mechanisms leading to their longevity in cancer patients. Better understanding of these mechanisms and using therapies to intercept these suppressive mechanisms are attractive strategies to prevent cancer resistance and recurrence.

2 In Vivo and In Vitro Tumor Models

Tumor microenvironment is complexed of neoplastic and non-neoplastic cellular and non-cellular components; all contribute to malignant constitution of cancers. Non-neoplastic cellular components consist of stromal, immune and mesenchymal stem cells. There are tremendous suggesting documents that tumoral non-neoplastic cells also encourage cancer initiation, progression and metastasis whose suppression or rearrangement can inhibit tumorigenesis. Recruiting in vivo and in vitro systems such as scaffold and matrix-based 3D systems -which were originally developed for regenerative medicine-, improved approaching these non-neoplastic components such as tumor stroma activity in progressed metastatic cancers. Moreover, pharmacodynamic and pharmacokinetic systems, including specific bio-material drug deliveries, to fight stromal cells or to reformat the microenvironment for tumor suppression, have been investigated. The impact of in vitro models such as 3D tumor models is so interesting in tumor biology.

2.1 PDX Models and Challenges

An in vivo model for the investigation of tumor microenvironment is patient-derived xenograft (PDX). Several characterized tumors-derived cell lines have been generated for cancer research. The first PDX model was introduced in the 1980s for providing a more accurate interpretation of laboratory results to clinical oncology [44–46]. The applications of PDX models utilizing implanted tumor fragments in immunodeficient mice have been increased in the recent years. PDX models with a wide variety of tumor histopathological types have particular and specific applications for the therapeutic purposes. Therefore having the most accurate model is essential in translational cancer research. However, the xenograft tumor cell lines do not accurately present the tumor microenvironment [47], as they typically never experience any in vitro conditions. We may significantly avoid any data misinterpretation while using PDX models by considering the potential gradual alterations of these models in tumor growth.

Some significant correlations have been documented in a number of cancers between genotype-phenotype (morpho-histopathological), gene expression pattern, and therapeutic responses between the original patient samples and PDX models grown over multiple passages [48–52]. However, these correlations and consistencies between them in response to antineoplastic treatment have not been confirmed at higher passages, resulting in no progress in interpretation of results. Human to murine transition of tumor-associated stromal tissue in the PDX models may interpret it [53].

Several quantitative methods have been used for evaluation the differences between sizes in xenograft tumor at a glance, but not from different time points yet. They include a number of Bayesian approaches for different treatment conditions [54–58]. However, no methods have been developed to evaluate longitudinal xenograft tumor growth information across multiple in vivo passages.

Some PDX models have been recently established for certain cancers utilizing new methods to include tumor size information on (in vivo) multi-passages, and on time periods beyond the murine hosts life span. A reduced time between passages has been observed as a common phenomenon among almost all cancers. These alterations are more likely to provide an accurate data interpretation of PDX models.

2.1.1　CTCs

CTCs are invaluable tools to study and monitor cancer progression. An important and relatively easy way to understand molecular mechanisms involved in tumor metastasis is to study tumor cells that are delaminated from primary tumor and circulate in blood system to reach other organs, which are called CTCs [1, 59]. Until recent years, most of the studies were focused on analysis of primary tumors, as well as therapeutic procedures that were pointed at eradication of cancer from the original site. However, when the primary tumors metastasize, almost no treatment is successful, and that is due to the lack of understanding of the events that follow, as well as the protective microenvironments where the secondary tumors reside. Now, taking advantage of new technologies it is possible to trace certain lineage of cells, and to scrutinize CTCs in terms of quantity and quality. This provides a plethora of information regarding events occurring inside tumors, providing new possibilities to fight cancer metastasis. Thus, studying and monitoring of CTCs have provided invaluable information, and seem to hold the key for future of cancer detection and treatment.

Several different methods have been developed to isolate CTCs from blood. Heterogeneity of CTCs has made it difficult to find a universal tumor marker isolation and enrichment. In general, approaches to isolate CTCs can be categorized to two groups; label-dependent and label-independent technologies. In first category, tumor cells are isolated based on their immunologic features like expression of certain markers, while in the second group morphological characteristics like size or density are used [60]. Each of these approaches have advantages and disadvantages that can affect diagnosis and consequently treatment of procedures. Hence, using an unbiased sensitive method is necessary for the field.

Label-dependent (LD) isolation of CTCs is based on detection of antigens that can be distinguished from that of blood cells. LD-based technologies are mostly based on detecting CTCs from carcinomas (cancers arising from epithelial tissue), therefore use epithelial specific markers such as EpCAM (epithelial cell surface adhesion molecule), or tumor specific markers such as HER2 [61]. LD-based methods have been used widely due to their specificity and significant improvement of capturing CTCs.

Although LD-based technologies are more specific, they can enrich certain subpopulation of CTCs, thus bias the analyses by missing cells that do not express that certain antigen. An important example is to miss mesenchymal cells when using epithelial markers like EpCAM for CTCs isolation. Carcinoma cells can undergo EMT that leads to loss of epithelial markers [2, 62]. Therefore, utilizing other markers to detect upregulated mesenchymal proteins is necessary for isolation of CTCs that have undergone EMT. Vimentin and N-cadherin are among upregulated markers in mesenchymal cells that could be used for detection of CTCs. However, because vimentin is also expressed in other normal blood cells, other analyses to distinguish tumor cells, like florescent in-situ hybridization (FISH) are required [63]. Plastin 3 is another marker that could be used for tumor cells that undergo EMT. It was identified in colorectal cancer patients that *PLS3* (plastin 3 gene) is not downregulated in CTCs that undergo EMT, while is not expressed in normal blood cells [64]. Thus, it could be used as a marker both for epithelial and mesenchymal CTCs. Cancer testis antigens (CTAs) are also among factors that can distinguish tumor cells in circulation. They are uniquely expressed in human germ line cells, and are also expressed in a variety of tumor cells. Thus, CTAs could be considered as most specific tumor markers with potential to detect CTCs [65–70]. Tumor specific markers are also obvious choices as markers for CTC detection. For instance, prostate-specific antigen (PSA) and prostate-specific membrane antigen (PSM) for prostate cancer, and HER2 are among largely characterized tumor specific markers [71, 72]. Of disadvantages of using specific markers for CTC detection could be case-specificity and lack of enough sensitivity for a wide range of stages among different cancer patients.

Another procedure to avoid bias in detecting CTCs is to use a combination of markers. In a study using a cocktail of antibodies, it was shown that detection of CTCs are largely improved compared to anti-EpCAM alone [73]. In this technique, the investigators used antibodies mixtures against a range of cell surface antigens including EpCAM, tumor-associated calcium signal transducer 2, c-MET, Folate-binding protein receptor, N-Cadherin, CD318, mesenchymal stem cell antigen, Her2, MUC-1, and EGFR, followed by detection using CEE-Enhanced (CE) fluorescence-labeled antibodies to capture CTCs. The latter is to avoid detecting only cytokeratin-positive tumor cells, which is another bias in detecting the captured cells [73].

Label-independent (LI) technologies for isolation of CTCs are based on morphological characteristics of tumor cells. Recently, several techniques have been developed in order to isolate CTCs in an unbiased manner. LD technologies are developed to specifically detect CTCs and to overcome the problem of missing a certain type of tumor cells, such as mesenchymal tumor cells, and to avoid using expensive and time-consuming LD techniques.

LID isolation methods are mainly based on size, density or microfluidic characteristic of CTCs. Of size-dependent methods ISET®, Parsortix and ScreenCell can be mentioned [74–76]. In ISET® (Isolation by Size of Epithelial Tumor cells) for instance, tumor cells are isolated by filtration as a result of their large size, following identification of trapped cells by immunohistochemical markers and quantitative real-time RT-PCR [77, 78]. However, some issues like damaging CTCs reduce the efficiency of this technology [79]. Density-based detection methods, like OncoQuickTM [80], and microfluidic characteristic-based method, like DFF-chip and JETTATM [81, 82], are among the other ones.

Detection of CTCs based on their size can be misleading due to the similarities to leukocytes. A new method called NELMEC (nano-electromechanical chip) is developed to detect both epithelial and mesenchymal CTCs. Detection is firstly based on size of single cells, and then on the analyses of the difference in membrane of the cells in order to WBCs from tumor cells. The different capacitance of CTCs and leukocytes is detected by nanograss (SiNG) electrodes [83].

Aside from capturing single CTCs, clustered CTCs are also of high clinical importance [84] and need to be properly detected. A microchip technology (the Cluster-Chip) is particularly developed for this purpose. This technique is independent from tumor-specific marker in capturing CTCs, and uses specialized bifurcating traps in conditions with low-shear stress, in order to preserve the viability and integrity of CTCs [85].

2.2 Microfluidic

Microfluidic technology can provide a suitable model system to study cancer biology. By combination of multiple controlled biophysical and biochemical microenvironment, together with high resolution real-time imaging, it has developed a useful platform to investigate complex behavior of cancer cells [86–88]. Accordingly, several microfluidic systems have been developed to investigate different aspects of cancer metastasis such as cancer cell migration and invasion, adhesion and extravasation [89–92].

2.3 Organoid Culture

To understand the biology of cancer and translate this knowledge into clinical treatment, preclinical cancer models are necessary to resemble the real situation in tumor and efficiently predict drug responses. However, this resemblance is rarely achieved using many of the widely-used cancer models [93].

Although having several advantages, cancer cell lines fall short of authentically representing the clinical status of cancer. Several widely-used cancer cell lines are originally derived from metastatic and fast growing tumor cells, therefore slowly growing, and many types of primary tumors are underrepresented in many of the studies that have used this system. In addition, in the process of obtaining cell lines, many subpopulations of tumor cells can be lost, due to selective new environment for certain types of cells. Therefore, cell lines lose tumor heterogeneity, and adapt to in vitro cultures. This leads to drastic shifts in gene expression patterns, consequently making cell lines not reliable for use in cancer biology research [94, 95].

To improve the status of cancer cells outside the human body PDTX have been developed, although not entirely satisfactory. PDTX are derived from implanting fresh tumor parts into immunocompromised animal. Basically, original tumor conditions are much better mimicked in this system compared to a plastic dish in case of cell lines, since they are maintained in physiological in vivo environment. PDTX have been developed for a variety of cancer types, and the biological stability and genetic diversity is considerably established [96–98]. However, there are several disadvantages for PDTX being used as a perfect preclinical model. One of the most important ones is that tumor take is not adequate, more efficiently are engrafting of aggressive tumors. In some cases, successful xenograft could be predictive as increased risk of disease recurrence [99]. In addition, interactions of tumor cells with host is not totally conserved, therefore similarity between the parental tumor and PDTX need to be analyzed in each case. And, the part of immune system is completely missing as xenografts are developed in immunocompromised animals [100]. Finally, utilization of animals is time consuming, much more expensive and ethically challenging. Thus, PDTX could not be widely accepted as substitutes for cell lines, considering features like high throughput drug screening [101]. These gaps in cell lines and PDTX may be improved by organoid cultures from primary tumors [102].

Extraordinary research has been focused on developing the use of human tissue surrogates in vitro in the recent years. Self-organization of epithelia of a certain tissue from corresponding adult stem cells happens when cells are embedded in a three-dimensional matrix. Much better than traditionally culturing cell lines, in organoid culture physiology of native epithelia is representing its origin. In cancer also, organoids derived from the tumor of a patient provides a valuable source to analyze biology of cancer and bring ex vivo assays to foster suitable treatment. Culturing patient-derived tumor cells as organoids (tumor organoids) results in preservation of genetic diversity [103]. Differentiation status and tumor heterogeneity and histoarchitecture can also be maintained in this system. Furthermore, patient-specific physiological changes like hypoxia and epigenetic marks have been retained [104]. To overcome one other weak points of cell line, which is rare normal cells derived from healthy tissue, organoids are also being developed from healthy tissue of the same individual [105]. Organoids can also derive from CTCs, as well as different cell type in different status of differentiation [106]. Organoid technology is one of the promising tools toward personalized treatment, and provide invaluable resource for bringing the gap between cancer genetics and clinical trial studies.

Organoid technology is also more powerful in combination with other new technologies such as CRISPR-Cas9 genome-editing system, and directed differentiation of stem cells. For instance, in a study using CRISPR the role of several different mutations has been scrutinized in developing colorectal cancer, introducing these mutations in organoids from normal human intestinal epithelium. It was shown that 'driver' pathway mutations, like APC, SMAD4, TP53, KRAS, and PIK3CA leads to stem cell maintenance in tumor microenvironment, while they are not enough for developing macrometastases and other molecular alterations such as chromosome instability are required [107]. On the other hand, organoid culture can provide a platform for directed differentiation in pluripotent stem cells. Exocrine pancreatic cells have been developed in order to study molecular mechanisms involved in pancreatic adenocarcinoma (PDAC). It was shown that specific mutation cause specific phenotype. KRAS or TP53 are two prevalently mutated genes in PDAC [104].

Organoids are promising tools to bring the gaps between cancer cell lines and PDTX. Although organoid culture has opened important doors towards understanding cancer biology, it lacks some of the advantages of other systems. Interaction of tumor cells with stroma and vasculature cannot be studied in organoids, as they are pure epithelial cultures. PDTX models are suitable for this purpose, as they are more physiologically relevant and allow analyses that require tumor-host interactions. On the other hand, drug screening can me more difficult in organoids compared to cell lines, as there are potentially complicating parameters in organoid culture system [102]. However, with recent advances organoids are considered as an invaluable tool to study several aspects of cancer progression, and combination of new technologies brings promise to transform this technology to be vastly used for personalized treatment and drug screening.

3   Concluding Remarks

One of the most promising ways to understand cancer biology is to study human-derived cancer models, where primary tumors are analyzed outside their host. On the other hand, precision or personalized medicine in cancer field is the future of cancer therapy. In this regard, preclinical tumor models that faithfully represent the tumor microenvironment are necessary for cancer research. However, a majority of the traditional models are not true representations of patients' tumors and may not accurately predict the clinical responses. As outlined above, the development of novel tumor models including 3D in vitro cultures called 'organoids' as well as cancer cell line and PDX models have provided useful platforms for studying tumor biology and therapeutic testing.

References

1. Valastyan S, Weinberg RA (2011) Tumor metastasis: molecular insights and evolving paradigms. Cell 147(2):275–292. doi:10.1016/j.cell.2011.09.024S0092-8674(11)01085-3
2. Nieto MA (2013) Epithelial plasticity: a common theme in embryonic and cancer cells. Science 342(6159):1234850. doi:10.1126/science.1234850342/6159/1234850
3. Nieto MA, Huang RY, Jackson RA, Thiery JP (2016) EMT: 2016. Cell 166(1):21–45. doi:10.1016/j.cell.2016.06.028
4. Ocana OH, Corcoles R, Fabra A, Moreno-Bueno G, Acloque H, Vega S et al (2012) Metastatic colonization requires the repression of the epithelial-mesenchymal transition inducer Prrx1. Cancer Cell 22(6):709–724. doi:10.1016/j.ccr.2012.10.012S1535-6108(12)00442-4
5. Tsai JH, Donaher JL, Murphy DA, Chau S, Yang J (2012) Spatiotemporal regulation of epithelial-mesenchymal transition is essential for squamous cell carcinoma metastasis. Cancer Cell 22(6):725–736. doi:10.1016/j.ccr.2012.09.022S1535-6108(12)00400-X
6. Brabletz T (2012) To differentiate or not: routes towards metastasis. Nat Rev Cancer 12(6):425–436. doi:10.1038/nrc3265nrc3265

7. Fazilaty H, Gardaneh M, Bahrami T, Salmaninejad A, Behnam B (2013) Crosstalk between breast cancer stem cells and metastatic niche: emerging molecular metastasis pathway? Tumour Biol 34(4):2019–2030. doi:10.1007/s13277-013-0831-y

8. Fazilaty H, Behnam B (2014) The perivascular niche governs an autoregulatory network to support breast cancer metastasis. Cell Biol Int 38(6):691–694. doi:10.1002/cbin.10261

9. Fazilaty H, Gardaneh M, Akbari P, Zekri A, Behnam B (2015) SLUG and SOX9 cooperatively regulate tumor initiating niche factors in breast cancer. Cancer Microenviron 9(1):71–74. doi:10.1007/s12307-015-0176-8

10. Fazilaty H, Mehdipour P (2014) Genetics of breast cancer bone metastasis: a sequential multistep pattern. Clin Exp Metastasis 31(5):595–612. doi:10.1007/s10585-014-9642-9

11. De Craene B, Berx G (2013) Regulatory networks defining EMT during cancer initiation and progression. Nat Rev Cancer 13(2):97–110. doi:10.1038/nrc3447nrc3447

12. Palucka AK, Coussens LM (2016) The basis of oncoimmunology. Cell 164(6):1233–1247. doi:10.1016/j.cell.2016.01.049

13. Hanahan D, Weinberg RA (2011) Hallmarks of cancer: the next generation. Cell 144(5):646–674. doi:10.1016/j.cell.2011.02.013

14. Bhatia A, Kumar Y (2016) Cancer stem cells and tumor immunoediting: putting two and two together. Expert Rev Clin Immunol 16:1–3 [Epub ahead of print]

15. Balic M, Williams A, Lin H, Datar R, Cote RJ (2013) Circulating tumor cells: from bench to bedside. Annu Rev Med 64:31–44. doi:10.1146/annurev-med-050311-163404

16. Majeti R, Chao MP, Alizadeh AA, Pang WW, Jaiswal S, Gibbs KD Jr, van Rooijen N, Weissman IL (2009) CD47 is an adverse prognostic factor and therapeutic antibody target on human acute myeloid leukemia stem cells. Cell 138(2):286–299. doi:10.1016/j.cell.2009.05.045

17. Kong F, Gao F, Li H, Liu H, Zhang Y, Zheng R, Zhang Y, Chen J, Li X, Liu G, Jia Y (2016) CD47: a potential immunotherapy target for eliminating cancer cells. Clin Transl Oncol. doi:10.1007/s12094-016-1489-x [Epub ahead of print]

18. Casey SC, Tong L, Li Y, Do R, Walz S, Fitzgerald KN, Gouw A, Baylot V, Guetegemann I, Eilers M, Felsher DW (2016) MYC regulates the antitumor immune response through CD47 and PD-L1. Science 352(6282):227–231

19. Zhang H, Lu H, Xiang L, Bullen JW, Zhang C, Samanta D, Gilkes DM, He J, Semenza GL (2015) HIF-1 regulates CD47 expression in breast cancer cells to promote evasion of phagocytosis and maintenance of cancer stem cells. Proc Natl Acad Sci U S A 112(45):E6215–E6223. doi:10.1073/pnas.1520032112

20. McCracken MN, Cha AC, Weissman IL (2015) Molecular pathways: activating T cells after cancer cell phagocytosis from blockade of CD47 "don't eat me" signals. Clin Cancer Res 21(16):3597–3601. doi:10.1158/1078-0432.CCR-14-2520

21. Rivera A, Fu X, Tao L, Zhang X (2015) Expression of mouse CD47 on human cancer cells profoundly increases tumor metastasis in murine models. BMC Cancer 15:964. doi:10.1186/s12885-015-1980-8

22. Chao MP, Alizadeh AA, Tang C, Myklebust JH, Varghese B, Gill S, Jan M, Cha AC, Chan CK, Tan BT, Park CY, Zhao F, Kohrt HE, Malumbres R, Briones J, Gascoyne RD, Lossos IS, Levy R, Weissman IL, Majeti R (2010) Anti-CD47 antibody synergizes with rituximab to promote phagocytosis and eradicate non-Hodgkin lymphoma. Cell 142(5):699–713. doi:10.1016/j.cell.2010.07.044

23. Liu J, Wang L, Zhao F, Tseng S, Narayanan C, Shura L, Willingham S, Howard M, Prohaska S, Volkmer J, Chao M, Weissman IL, Majeti R (2015) Pre-clinical development of a humanized anti-CD47 antibody with anti-cancer therapeutic potential. PLoS One 10(9), e0137345. doi:10.1371/journal.pone.0137345

24. Hatherley D, Lea SM, Johnson S, Barclay AN (2013) Structures of CD200/CD200 receptor family and implications for topology, regulation, and evolution. Structure 21(5):820–832. doi:10.1016/j.str.2013.03.008

25. Jenmalm MC, Cherwinski H, Bowman EP, Phillips JH, Sedgwick JD (2006) Regulation of myeloid cell function through the CD200 receptor. J Immunol 176(1):191–199

26. Kawasaki BT, Farrar WL (2008) Cancer stem cells, CD200 and immunoevasion. Trends Immunol 29(10):464–468. doi:10.1016/j.it.2008.07.005

27. Siva A, Xin H, Qin F, Oltean D, Bowdish KS, Kretz-Rommel A (2008) Immune modulation by melanoma and ovarian tumor cells through expression of the immunosuppressive molecule CD200. Cancer Immunol Immunother 57(7):987–996

28. Gorczynski RM, Chen Z, Hu J, Kai Y, Lei J (2001) Evidence of a role for CD200 in regulation of immune rejection of leukaemic tumour cells in C57BL/6 mice. Clin Exp Immunol 126(2):220–229

29. Kawasaki BT, Mistree T, Hurt EM, Kalathur M, Farrar WL (2007) Co-expression of the tolleragenic glycoprotein, CD200, with markers for cancer stem cells. Biochem Biophys Res Commun 364(4):778–782

30. Kretz-Rommel A, Qin F, Dakappagari N, Cofiell R, Faas SJ, Bowdish KS (2008) Blockade of CD200 in the presence or absence of antibody effector function: implications for anti-CD200 therapy. J Immunol 180(2):699–705

31. Pan Q, Li Q, Liu S, Ning N, Zhang X, Xu Y, Chang AE, Wicha MS (2015) Concise review: targeting cancer stem cells using immunologic approaches. Stem Cells 33(7):2085–2092. doi:10.1002/stem.2039

32. Jin L, Hope KJ, Zhai Q, Smadja-Joffe F, Dick JE (2006) Targeting of CD44 eradicates human acute myeloid leukemic stem cells. Nat Med 12(10):1167–1174

33. Takaishi S, Okumura T, Tu S, Wang SS, Shibata W, Vigneshwaran R, Gordon SA, Shimada Y, Wang TC (2009) Identification of gastric cancer stem cells using the cell surface marker CD44. Stem Cells 27(5):1006–1020. doi:10.1002/stem.30

34. Du L, Wang H, He L, Zhang J, Ni B, Wang X, Jin H, Cahuzac N, Mehrpour M, Lu Y, Chen Q (2008) CD44 is of functional importance for colorectal cancer stem cells. Clin Cancer Res 14(21):6751–6760. doi:10.1158/1078-0432.CCR-08-1034

35. Jaggupilli A, Elkord E (2012) Significance of CD44 and CD24 as cancer stem cell markers: an enduring ambiguity. Clin Dev Immunol 2012:708036. doi:10.1155/2012/708036

36. Chen S, Song X, Chen Z, Li X, Li M, Liu H, Li J (2013) CD133 expression and the prognosis of colorectal cancer: a systematic review and meta-analysis. PLoS One 8(2), e56380. doi:10.1371/journal.pone.0056380

37. Huang J, Li C, Wang Y, Lv H, Guo Y, Dai H, Wicha MS, Chang AE, Li Q (2013) Cytokine-induced killer (CIK) cells bound with anti-CD3/anti-CD133 bispecific antibodies target CD133high cancer stem cells in vitro and in vivo. Clin Immunol 149(1):156–168. doi:10.1016/j.clim.2013.07.006

38. Shipitsin M, Campbell LL, Argani P, Weremowicz S, Bloushtain-Qimron N, Yao J, Nikolskaya T, Serebryiskaya T, Beroukhim R, Hu M, Halushka MK, Sukumar S, Parker LM, Anderson KS, Harris LN, Garber JE, Richardson AL, Schnitt SJ, Nikolsky Y, Gelman RS, Polyak K (2007) Molecular definition of breast tumor heterogeneity. Cancer Cell 11(3):259–273

39. Lottaz C, Beier D, Meyer K, Kumar P, Hermann A, Schwarz J, Junker M, Oefner PJ, Bogdahn U, Wischhusen J, Spang R, Storch A, Beier CP (2010) Transcriptional profiles of CD133+ and CD133- glioblastoma-derived cancer stem cell lines suggest different cells of origin. Cancer Res 70(5):2030–2040. doi:10.1158/0008-5472.CAN-09-1707

40. Todaro M, Alea MP, Di Stefano AB, Cammareri P, Vermeulen L, Iovino F, Tripodo C, Russo A, Gulotta G, Medema JP, Stassi G (2007) Colon cancer stem cells dictate tumor growth and resist cell death by production of interleukin-4. Cell Stem Cell 1(4):389–402. doi:10.1016/j.stem.2007.08.001

41. Olver S, Groves P, Buttigieg K, Morris ES, Janas ML, Kelso A, Kienzle N (2006) Tumor-derived interleukin-4 reduces tumor clearance and deviates the cytokine and granzyme profile of tumor-induced CD8+ T cells. Cancer Res 66(1):571–580

42. Rutella S, Danese S, Leone G (2006) Tolerogenic dendritic cells: cytokine modulation comes of age. Blood 108(5):1435–1440

43. Mantovani A, Sozzani S, Locati M, Allavena P, Sica A (2002) Macrophage polarization: tumor-associated macrophages as a paradigm for polarized M2 mononuclear phagocytes. Trends Immunol 23(11):549–555

44. Fiebig HH, Neumann HA, Henss H, Koch H, Kaiser D, Arnold H (1985) Development of three human small cell lung cancer models in nude mice. Recent Results Cancer Res 97:77–86
45. Povlsen CO, Rygaard J (1972) Heterotransplantation of human epidermoid carcinomas to the mouse mutant nude. Acta Pathol Microbiol Scand A 80:713–717
46. Braakhuis BJ, Sneeuwloper G, Snow GB (1984) The potential of the nude mouse xenograft model for the study of head and neck cancer. Arch Otorhinolaryngol 239:69–79
47. Johnson JI, Decker S, Zaharevitz D, Rubinstein LV, Venditti JM, Schepartz S, Kalyandrug S, Christian M, Arbuck S, Hollingshead M, Sausville EA (2001) Relationships between drug activity in NCI preclinical in vitro and in vivo models and early clinical trials. Br J Cancer 84:1424–1431
48. Fichtner I, Rolff J, Soong R, Hoffmann J, Hammer S, Sommer A, Becker M, Merk J (2008) Establishment of patient- derived non-small cell lung cancer xenografts as models for the identification of predictive biomarkers. Clin Cancer Res 14:6456–6468
49. DeRose YS, Wang G, Lin YC, Bernard PS, Buys SS, Ebbert MT, Factor R, Matsen C, Milash BA, Nelson E, Neumayer L, Randall RL, Stijleman IJ et al (2011) Tumor grafts derived from women with breast cancer authentically reflect tumor pathology, growth, metastasis and disease outcomes. Nat Med 17:1514–1520
50. Zhang X, Claerhout S, Prat A, Dobrolecki LE, Petrovic I, Lai Q, Landis MD, Wiechmann L, Schiff R, Giuliano M, Wong H, Fuqua SW, Contreras A et al (2013) A renewable tissue resource of phenotypically stable, biologically and ethnically diverse, patient-derived human breast cancer xenograft models. Cancer Res 73:4885–4897
51. Hidalgo M, Amant F, Biankin AV, Budinska E, Byrne AT, Caldas C, Clarke RB, de Jong S, Jonkers J, Maelandsmo GM, Roman-Roman S, Seoane J, Trusolino L et al (2014) Patient-derived xenograft models: an emerging platform for translational cancer research. Cancer Discov 4:998–1013
52. Keysar SB, Astling DP, Anderson RT, Vogler BW, Bowles DW, Morton JJ, Paylor JJ, Glogowska MJ, Le PN, Eagles-Soukup JR, Kako SL, Takimoto SM, Sehrt DB et al (2013) A patient tumor transplant model of squamous cell cancer identifies PI3K inhibitors as candidate therapeutics in defined molecular bins. Mol Oncol 7:776–790
53. Reyal F, Guyader C, Decraene C, Lucchesi C, Auger N, Assayag F, De Plater L, Gentien D, Poupon MF, Cottu P, De Cremoux P, Gestraud P, Vincent-Salomon A et al (2012) Molecular profiling of patient-derived breast cancer xenografts. Breast Cancer Res 14:R11
54. Mann HB, Whitney DR (1947) On a test of whether one of two random variables is stochastically larger than the other. Ann Math Stat 18(1):50–60
55. Anscombe FJ (1948) The validity of comparative experiments. J R Stat Soc Ser A 111:181–211
56. Scheffé H (1999) The analysis of variance. Wiley, New York, NY
57. Milton F (1937) The use of ranks to avoid the assumption of normality implicit in the analysis of variance. J Am Stat Assoc 32:675–701
58. Laird NM, Ware JH (1982) Random-effects models for longitudinal data. Biometrics 38:963–974
59. Chaffer CL, Weinberg RA (2011) A perspective on cancer cell metastasis. Science 331(6024):1559–1564. doi:10.1126/science.1203543331/6024/1559
60. Broersen LH, van Pelt GW, Tollenaar RA, Mesker WE (2014) Clinical application of circulating tumor cells in breast cancer. Cell Oncol (Dordr) 37(1):9–15. doi:10.1007/s13402-013-0160-6
61. Pantel K, Alix-Panabières C (2013) Real-time liquid biopsy in cancer patients: fact or fiction? Cancer Res 73(21):6384–6388
62. Kalluri R, Weinberg RA (2009) The basics of epithelial-mesenchymal transition. J Clin Invest 119(6):1420–1428. doi:10.1172/JCI3910439104
63. Bednarz N, Eltze E, Semjonow A, Rink M, Andreas A, Mulder L et al (2010) BRCA1 loss preexisting in small subpopulations of prostate cancer is associated with advanced disease and metastatic spread to lymph nodes and peripheral blood. Clin Cancer Res 16(13):3340–3348
64. Yokobori T, Iinuma H, Shimamura T, Imoto S, Sugimachi K, Ishii H et al (2013) Plastin3 is a novel marker for circulating tumor cells undergoing the epithelial–mesenchymal transition and is associated with colorectal cancer prognosis. Cancer Res 73(7):2059–2069

65. Novikov D, Belova T, Plekhanova E, Yanchenko O, Novikov V (2012) Early detection of cancer/testis mRNAs in tumor cells circulating in the peripheral blood of colorectal cancer patients. Mol Biol 46(5):687–692

66. Gumireddy K, Li A, Chang DH, Liu Q, Kossenkov AV, Yan J et al (2015) AKAP4 is a circulating biomarker for non-small cell lung cancer. Oncotarget 6(19):17637–17647. doi:10.18632/oncotarget.3946

67. Behnam B, Chahlavi A, Pattisapu J, Wolfe J (2009) TSGA10 is specifically expressed in astrocyte and over-expressed in brain tumors. Avicenna J Med Biotechnol 1(3):161

68. Simpson AJ, Caballero OL, Jungbluth A, Chen Y-T, Old LJ (2005) Cancer/testis antigens, gametogenesis and cancer. Nat Rev Cancer 5(8):615–625

69. Behnam B, Conti V, Puliti A, Wolfe J (2006) TSGA10 expression during embryogenesis and neural development in parallel of spermatogenesis and malignancies. Dev Biol 295(1):466

70. Behnam B, Modarressi MH, Conti V, Taylor KE, Puliti A, Wolfe J (2006) Expression of Tsga10 sperm tail protein in embryogenesis and neural development: from cilium to cell division. Biochem Biophys Res Commun 344(4):1102–1110

71. Israeli RS, Miller WH, Su SL, Powell CT, Fair WR, Samadi DS et al (1994) Sensitive nested reverse transcription polymerase chain reaction detection of circulating prostatic tumor cells: comparison of prostate-specific membrane antigen and prostate-specific antigen-based assays. Cancer Res 54(24):6306–6310

72. Bidard F-C, Fehm T, Ignatiadis M, Smerage JB, Alix-Panabières C, Janni W et al (2013) Clinical application of circulating tumor cells in breast cancer: overview of the current interventional trials. Cancer Metastasis Rev 32(1-2):179–188

73. Mikolajczyk SD, Millar LS, Tsinberg P, Coutts SM, Zomorrodi M, Pham T et al (2011) Detection of EpCAM-negative and cytokeratin-negative circulating tumor cells in peripheral blood. J Oncol 2011:252361. doi:10.1155/2011/252361

74. Lin HK, Zheng S, Williams AJ, Balic M, Groshen S, Scher HI et al (2010) Portable filter-based microdevice for detection and characterization of circulating tumor cells. Clin Cancer Res 16(20):5011–5018. doi:10.1158/1078-0432.CCR-10-11051078-0432.CCR-10-1105

75. Freidin MB, Tay A, Freydina DV, Chudasama D, Nicholson AG, Rice A et al (2014) An assessment of diagnostic performance of a filter-based antibody-independent peripheral blood circulating tumour cell capture paired with cytomorphologic criteria for the diagnosis of cancer. Lung Cancer 85(2):182–185. doi:10.1016/j.lungcan.2014.05.017S0169-5002(14)00245-1

76. Kulemann B, Pitman MB, Liss AS, Valsangkar N, Fernandez-Del Castillo C, Lillemoe KD et al (2015) Circulating tumor cells found in patients with localized and advanced pancreatic cancer. Pancreas 44(4):547–550. doi:10.1097/MPA.0000000000000324

77. Vona G, Sabile A, Louha M, Sitruk V, Romana S, Schutze K et al (2000) Isolation by size of epithelial tumor cells: a new method for the immunomorphological and molecular characterization of circulating tumor cells. Am J Pathol 156(1):57–63. doi:10.1016/S0002-9440(10)64706-2

78. De Giorgi V, Pinzani P, Salvianti F, Panelos J, Paglierani M, Janowska A et al (2010) Application of a filtration- and isolation-by-size technique for the detection of circulating tumor cells in cutaneous melanoma. J Invest Dermatol 130(10):2440–2447. doi:10.1038/jid.2010.141jid2010141

79. Warkiani ME, Khoo BL, Wu L, Tay AK, Bhagat AA, Han J et al (2016) Ultra-fast, label-free isolation of circulating tumor cells from blood using spiral microfluidics. Nat Protoc 11(1):134–148. doi:10.1038/nprot.2016.003

80. Muller V, Stahmann N, Riethdorf S, Rau T, Zabel T, Goetz A et al (2005) Circulating tumor cells in breast cancer: correlation to bone marrow micrometastases, heterogeneous response to systemic therapy and low proliferative activity. Clin Cancer Res 11(10):3678–3685. doi:10.1158/1078-0432.CCR-04-2469

81. Riahi R, Gogoi P, Sepehri S, Zhou Y, Handique K, Godsey J et al (2014) A novel microchannel-based device to capture and analyze circulating tumor cells (CTCs) of breast cancer. Int J Oncol 44(6):1870–1878. doi:10.3892/ijo.2014.2353

82. Hou HW, Warkiani ME, Khoo BL, Li ZR, Soo RA, Tan DS et al (2013) Isolation and retrieval of circulating tumor cells using centrifugal forces. Sci Rep 3:1259. doi:10.1038/srep01259
83. Hosseini SA, Abdolahad M, Zanganeh S, Dahmardeh M, Gharooni M, Abiri H et al (2016) Nanoelectromechanical chip (NELMEC) combination of nanoelectronics and microfluidics to diagnose epithelial and mesenchymal circulating tumor cells from leukocytes. Small 12(7):883–891. doi:10.1002/smll.201502808
84. Aceto N, Bardia A, Miyamoto DT, Donaldson MC, Wittner BS, Spencer JA et al (2014) Circulating tumor cell clusters are oligoclonal precursors of breast cancer metastasis. Cell 158(5):1110–1122. doi:10.1016/j.cell.2014.07.013S0092-8674(14)00927-1
85. Sarioglu AF, Aceto N, Kojic N, Donaldson MC, Zeinali M, Hamza B et al (2015) A microfluidic device for label-free, physical capture of circulating tumor cell clusters. Nat Methods 12(7):685–691. doi:10.1038/nmeth.3404
86. Nie FQ, Yamada M, Kobayashi J, Yamato M, Kikuchi A, Okano T (2007) On-chip cell migration assay using microfluidic channels. Biomaterials 28(27):4017–4022. doi:10.1016/j.biomaterials.2007.05.037
87. Yang K, Han S, Shin Y, Ko E, Kim J, Park KI et al (2013) A microfluidic array for quantitative analysis of human neural stem cell self-renewal and differentiation in three-dimensional hypoxic microenvironment. Biomaterials 34(28):6607–6614. doi:10.1016/j.biomaterials.2013.05.067S0142-9612(13)00659-5
88. Chung S, Sudo R, Mack PJ, Wan CR, Vickerman V, Kamm RD (2009) Cell migration into scaffolds under co-culture conditions in a microfluidic platform. Lab Chip 9(2):269–275. doi:10.1039/b807585a
89. Haessler U, Teo JC, Foretay D, Renaud P, Swartz MA (2012) Migration dynamics of breast cancer cells in a tunable 3D interstitial flow chamber. Integr Biol (Camb) 4(4):401–409. doi:10.1039/c1ib00128k
90. Liu T, Li C, Li H, Zeng S, Qin J, Lin B (2009) A microfluidic device for characterizing the invasion of cancer cells in 3-D matrix. Electrophoresis 30(24):4285–4291. doi:10.1002/elps.200900289
91. Song JW, Cavnar SP, Walker AC, Luker KE, Gupta M, Tung YC et al (2009) Microfluidic endothelium for studying the intravascular adhesion of metastatic breast cancer cells. PLoS One 4(6), e5756. doi:10.1371/journal.pone.0005756
92. Jeon JS, Zervantonakis IK, Chung S, Kamm RD, Charest JL (2013) In vitro model of tumor cell extravasation. PLoS One 8(2), e56910. doi:10.1371/journal.pone.0056910PONE-D-12-35719
93. Kamb A (2005) What's wrong with our cancer models? Nat Rev Drug Discov 4(2):161–165. doi:10.1038/nrd1635
94. Masters JR (2000) Human cancer cell lines: fact and fantasy. Nat Rev Mol Cell Biol 1(3):233–236. doi:10.1038/35043102
95. van Staveren WC, Solis DY, Hebrant A, Detours V, Dumont JE, Maenhaut C (2009) Human cancer cell lines: experimental models for cancer cells in situ? For cancer stem cells? Biochim Biophys Acta 1795(2):92–103. doi:10.1016/j.bbcan.2008.12.004S0304-419X(08)00079-6
96. Tentler JJ, Tan AC, Weekes CD, Jimeno A, Leong S, Pitts TM et al (2012) Patient-derived tumour xenografts as models for oncology drug development. Nat Rev Clin Oncol 9(6):338–350. doi:10.1038/nrclinonc.2012.61
97. Daniel VC, Marchionni L, Hierman JS, Rhodes JT, Devereux WL, Rudin CM et al (2009) A primary xenograft model of small-cell lung cancer reveals irreversible changes in gene expression imposed by culture in vitro. Cancer Res 69(8):3364–3373. doi:10.1158/0008-5472.CAN-08-42100008-5472.CAN-08-4210
98. Jin K, Teng L, Shen Y, He K, Xu Z, Li G (2010) Patient-derived human tumour tissue xenografts in immunodeficient mice: a systematic review. Clin Transl Oncol 12(7):473–480. doi:10.1007/s12094-010-0540-6

99. John T, Kohler D, Pintilie M, Yanagawa N, Pham NA, Li M et al (2011) The ability to form primary tumor xenografts is predictive of increased risk of disease recurrence in early-stage non-small cell lung cancer. Clin Cancer Res 17(1):134–141. doi:10.1158/1078-0432.CCR-10-22241078-0432.CCR-10-2224

100. Caponigro G, Sellers WR (2011) Advances in the preclinical testing of cancer therapeutic hypotheses. Nat Rev Drug Discov 10(3):179–187. doi:10.1038/nrd3385nrd3385

101. Bernards R (2012) A missing link in genotype-directed cancer therapy. Cell 151(3):465–468. doi:10.1016/j.cell.2012.10.014S0092-8674(12)01228-7

102. Sachs N, Clevers H (2014) Organoid cultures for the analysis of cancer phenotypes. Curr Opin Genet Dev 24:68–73. doi:10.1016/j.gde.2013.11.012S0959-437X(13)00161-5

103. Weeber F, van de Wetering M, Hoogstraat M, Dijkstra KK, Krijgsman O, Kuilman T et al (2015) Preserved genetic diversity in organoids cultured from biopsies of human colorectal cancer metastases. Proc Natl Acad Sci U S A 112(43):13308–13311. doi:10.1073/pnas.15166891121516689112

104. Huang L, Holtzinger A, Jagan I, BeGora M, Lohse I, Ngai N et al (2015) Ductal pancreatic cancer modeling and drug screening using human pluripotent stem cell- and patient-derived tumor organoids. Nat Med 21(11):1364–1371. doi:10.1038/nm.3973nm.3973

105. van de Wetering M, Francies HE, Francis JM, Bounova G, Iorio F, Pronk A et al (2015) Prospective derivation of a living organoid biobank of colorectal cancer patients. Cell 161(4):933–945. doi:10.1016/j.cell.2015.03.053

106. Drost J, Karthaus WR, Gao D, Driehuis E, Sawyers CL, Chen Y et al (2016) Organoid culture systems for prostate epithelial and cancer tissue. Nat Protoc 11(2):347–358. doi:10.1038/nprot.2016.006nprot.2016.006

107. Matano M, Date S, Shimokawa M, Takano A, Fujii M, Ohta Y et al (2015) Modeling colorectal cancer using CRISPR-Cas9-mediated engineering of human intestinal organoids. Nat Med 21(3):256–262. doi:10.1038/nm.3802

108. Noman MZ, Messai Y, Muret J, Hasmim M, Chouaib S (2014) Crosstalk between CTC, immune system and hypoxic tumor microenvironment. Cancer Microenviron 7(3):153–160. doi:10.1007/s12307-014-0157-3

Printed in the United States
By Bookmasters